Second Edition

Physical Therapy Documentation

From Examination to Outcome

Second Edition

Physical Therapy Documentation

From Examination to Outcome

Mia L. Erickson, PT, EdD, CHT, ATC
Associate Professor and Co-Academic Coordinator of Clinical Education
Division of Physical Therapy
West Virginia University School of Medicine
Morgantown, West Virginia

Ralph R. Utzman, PT, MPH, PhD
Associate Professor and Co-Academic Coordinator of Clinical Education
Division of Physical Therapy
West Virginia University School of Medicine
Morgantown, West Virginia

Rebecca McKnight, PT, MS
Co-Owner
Reach Consulting
Powersite, Missouri

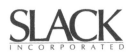

SLACK
INCORPORATED

www.Healio.com/books

ISBN: 978-1-61711-251-5

Copyright © 2014 by SLACK Incorporated

Instructors: *The Physical Therapy Documentation: From Examination to Outcome, Second Edition Instructor's Manual* is also available from SLACK Incorporated. Don't miss this important companion to *Physical Therapy Documentation: From Examination to Outcome, Second Edition.* To obtain the Instructor's Manual, please visit http://www.efacultylounge.com

The procedures and practices described in this publication should be implemented in a manner consistent with the professional standards set for the circumstances that apply in each specific situation. Every effort has been made to confirm the accuracy of the information presented and to correctly relate generally accepted practices. The authors, editors, and publisher cannot accept responsibility for errors or exclusions or for the outcome of the material presented herein. There is no expressed or implied warranty of this book or information imparted by it. Care has been taken to ensure that drug selection and dosages are in accordance with currently accepted/recommended practice. Off-label uses of drugs may be discussed. Due to continuing research, changes in government policy and regulations, and various effects of drug reactions and interactions, it is recommended that the reader carefully review all materials and literature provided for each drug, especially those that are new or not frequently used. Some drugs or devices in this publication have clearance for use in a restricted research setting by the Food and Drug and Administration or FDA. Each professional should determine the FDA status of any drug or device prior to use in their practice.

Any review or mention of specific companies or products is not intended as an endorsement by the author or publisher.

SLACK Incorporated uses a review process to evaluate submitted material. Prior to publication, educators or clinicians provide important feedback on the content that we publish. We welcome feedback on this work.

Published by: SLACK Incorporated
                 6900 Grove Road
                 Thorofare, NJ 08086 USA
                 Telephone: 856-848-1000
                 Fax: 856-848-6091
                 www.Healio.com/books

Contact SLACK Incorporated for more information about other books in this field or about the availability of our books from distributors outside the United States.

Library of Congress Cataloging-in-Publication Data

    Erickson, Mia L., author.
    Physical therapy documentation : from examination to outcome / Mia Erickson, Ralph Utzman, Rebecca McKnight. -- Second edition.
        p. ; cm.
    Includes bibliographical references and index.
    ISBN 978-1-61711-251-5 (alk. paper)
    I. Utzman, Ralph, 1966- author. II. McKnight, Rebecca, 1969- author. III. Title.
    [DNLM: 1. Medical Records. 2. Physical Therapy Specialty--organization & administration. 3. Forms and Records Control. WB 460]
    RM705
    615.8'2--dc23

                            2013032849

For permission to reprint material in another publication, contact SLACK Incorporated. Authorization to photocopy items for internal, personal, or academic use is granted by SLACK Incorporated provided that the appropriate fee is paid directly to Copyright Clearance Center. Prior to photocopying items, please contact the Copyright Clearance Center at 222 Rosewood Drive, Danvers, MA 01923 USA; phone: 978-750-8400; website: www.copyright.com; email: info@copyright.com

Printed in the United States of America.

Last digit is print number: 10 9 8 7 6 5 4

Contents

Instructors: *The Physical Therapy Documentation: From Examination to Outcome, Second Edition Instructor's Manual* is also available from SLACK Incorporated. Don't miss this important companion to *Physical Therapy Documentation: From Examination to Outcome, Second Edition.* To obtain the Instructor's Manual, please visit http://www.efacultylounge.com

Acknowledgments

I would like to say thank you to Ralph and Becky for continuing to see the need for this text and for supporting this project. Thank you also for your countless hours of work and contributions. I am also grateful to all the students who have used this text and allowed me to see areas where we needed to improve. This has kept me accountable for providing a high-quality product and striving to make it the best textbook for documentation available. To my family, thank you for allowing me the hours to make this happen.

Mia L. Erickson, PT, EdD, CHT, ATC

First, I would like to thank Mia and Becky for inviting me to participate in this wonderful project. It has been a joy to work with and learn from you both. I would also like to thank Jane Pertko, PT, GCS, who taught my first documentation class in physical therapy school. She taught the importance of documenting the PT thought process in a clear, complete, and concise way, which is more important now than ever. Finally, I would like to thank my wife, Donna, and our kids (Ryan, Nathan, Logan, and Gretchan) for their love and support.

Ralph R. Utzman, PT, MPH, PhD

ABOUT THE AUTHORS

Mia L. Erickson, PT, EdD, CHT, ATC is an associate professor and co-Academic Coordinator of Clinical Education in the Division of Physical Therapy at the West Virginia University School of Medicine. Mia holds a Bachelor's Degree from West Virginia University in Secondary Education and a Master's of Science Degree in Physical Therapy from the University of Indianapolis. She earned her doctor of education degree with emphasis in Curriculum and Instruction from West Virginia University. Her clinical practice is in the area of hand and upper extremity rehabilitation.

Ralph R. Utzman, PT, MPH, PhD is an associate professor and co-Academic Coordinator of Clinical Education in the Division of Physical Therapy at the West Virginia University School of Medicine. He holds a Bachelor's Degree in Physical Therapy and a master's degree in Public Health from West Virginia University, and a PhD in Health Related Sciences from the MCV Campus of Virginia Commonwealth University. His current clinical practice focuses on patients with vestibular disorders and Parkinson's disease. He teaches in the areas of professional practice roles, practice administration, and clinical skills.

Rebecca McKnight, PT, MS received her Bachelor's of Science degree in Physical Therapy from St. Louis University in 1992 and her post-professional Master's of Science degree from Rocky Mountain University of Health Professions in 1999. Rebecca taught in the Physical Therapist Assistant Program at Ozarks Technical Community College in Springfield, MO from 1997 to 2011. Nine of those years she served as Program Director. Currently Rebecca provides consultation related to curriculum design, development, and assessment through her company Reach Consulting. Rebecca is an active member of the American Physical Therapy Association, primarily within the Education Section.

PREFACE

Thank you for choosing the second edition of *Physical Therapy Documentation: From Examination to Outcome*. We are excited to provide you with an up-to-date tool for clinical documentation in physical therapy. This book serves mainly as a primer for learning to navigate the medical record and to construct relevant documentation necessary for survival in the current health care environment. It is laid out to present the basics of documentation, such as various formats, rules for writing in medical records, and reasons for documenting. However, the difference between this text and others is that the mechanics of writing are taught in such a way that basic documentation elements are blended with contemporary concepts.

Serving as a foundation, the International Classification of Functioning, Disabilities, and Health (ICF) disablement framework is used to emphasize the integration of function, results of physical therapy interventions, and patient improvement. Building on this, we have blended requirements for current documentation such as showing the unique skills we provide patients and describing why interventions are medically necessary.

While we continue with the use of the subjective, objective, assessment, and plan (SOAP) structure, we have emphasized the need for high-quality content within each section. We believe that using this structure for teaching the basics of documentation provides beginners with the knowledge and skills for adapting the documentation content into either paper or electronic records.

One more advanced feature of this text that will appeal to clinicians with all levels of experience is the integration of evidence-based practice into documentation. For example, we have blended the use of measurement properties of common tests and measures into goal writing and assessing change and outcome. More experienced clinicians will also benefit from the information to improving documentation quality in the areas of skilled care and medical necessity.

In addition, we provide the reader with examples and practice problems ranging from simple to complex. These examples and problems come from various practice settings and allow the user to develop basic skills and then transition to developing a plan of care, developing progress reports, and writing discharge documentation. Instructors can also benefit from the Instructor's Manual.

We are happy to provide this to our audience and students of documentation who will carry these concepts into clinical practice. Enjoy.

Chapter 1

Overview of Disablement

Mia L. Erickson, PT, EdD, CHT, ATC

CHAPTER OUTLINE

Disablement Frameworks
   International Classification of Functioning, Disability, and Health
   The Nagi Disablement Framework
   The National Center for Medical Rehabilitation Research Classification Scheme for Disability Terminology
Disablement and Physical Therapy
Disablement and Documentation
Summary

CHAPTER OBJECTIVES

Upon completion of this chapter, the reader will be able to:
1. Compare and contrast historical and contemporary disablement models.
2. Discuss the need for standard disablement concepts in patient care, health policy, and research.
3. List 3 disablement frameworks, or models.
4. Compare and contrast ICF and Nagi framework terminology.
5. Differentiate between body functions/structures, activities and participation, and contextual factors.
6. Differentiate between positive factors and negative factors.
7. Describe the components and purpose of the WHO-FIC.
8. Describe core set and its application for physical therapists.
9. Examine the integration of disablement in physical therapy practice.
10. List ways to integrate disablement concepts into documentation.

Erickson ML, Utzman RR, McKnight R. *Physical Therapy Documentation:*
From Examination to Outcome, Second Edition (pp 1-12).
© 2014 SLACK Incorporated.

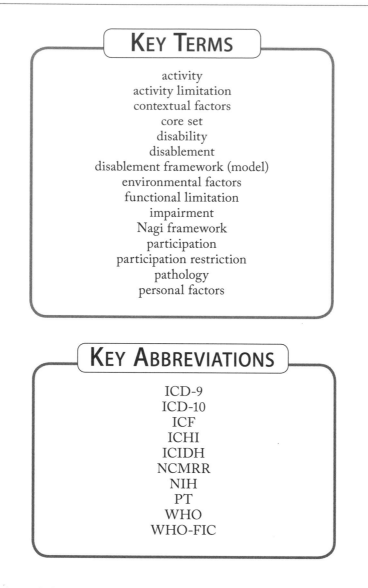

KEY TERMS

activity
activity limitation
contextual factors
core set
disability
disablement
disablement framework (model)
environmental factors
functional limitation
impairment
Nagi framework
participation
participation restriction
pathology
personal factors

KEY ABBREVIATIONS

ICD-9
ICD-10
ICF
ICHI
ICIDH
NCMRR
NIH
PT
WHO
WHO-FIC

The traditional approach to defining a person's state of health comes from the biomedical model where health means free of, or absent from, disease.[1,2] Under this model, disease means there is an abnormality within the body that gives rise to signs and symptoms.[2] Treating and curing the disease is often a primary focus of health care in this biomedical model. Additionally, in traditional medical models, there is often little emphasis on how the disease, or health condition, affects the individual's ability to participate in society. A more contemporary meaning of health goes beyond the mere presence or absence of disease or injury. The World Health Organization (WHO) defined health as a state where there is complete physical, mental, and social well-being and not merely the absence of disease or infirmity.[3] A person's health, or state of health, is also highly individualized and can *only* be defined in terms of the individual's functional goals and expectations to participate in society.[4]

As health is highly individualized, so are the effects of disease. The presence of a disease or illness does not directly correlate with the inability to perform self-care skills, function in the home environment, attain gainful employment,

Example 1-1. Effects of Disease on Function—Cerebrovascular Accident

Think about the following 2 patients who have had a cerebrovascular accident (CVA). Patient A had a small middle carotid artery bleed with little motor and sensory loss. One year later, he is able to safely perform all mobility activities (eg, walking around the house and the community), self- and home-care activities, and some higher-level thinking activities, thereby allowing him to work in a part-time job. Patient B, with the same diagnosis of CVA, had a massive bleed and did not have rapid access to adequate medical care. His clinical presentation was more complex and the outcome was much less favorable. This patient requires 24-hour care, assistance to move in and out of bed, and a wheelchair for all mobility.

Example 1-2. Effects of Disease on Function—Multiple Sclerosis

Now consider the medical diagnosis multiple sclerosis (MS). Miss A is a 35-year-old woman who was diagnosed with MS 1 year ago. She has been taking a new drug that has decreased the severity and frequency of her exacerbations. Miss A lives alone, drives, works at a bank, and plays recreational golf. She is very functional and independent within her environment. Now consider Miss B. She is a 56-year-old woman who was diagnosed with MS 12 years ago. Since the time of the diagnosis, she has lost the ability to drive, ambulate community distances, and perform her normal work duties.

---

or participate in community or social activities. In addition, the same medical diagnosis can have different effects on different people. It is often the severity of the illness and/or the disease consequences that most influence the individual's functional capacity (see Examples).

After looking at these examples, it should be apparent that presence of disease alone should not be the sole basis for determining a patient's functional capabilities. Because of the individual nature of health, it is important for health care providers to consider the consequence(s) of any health condition for every patient encountered. These consequences can dramatically influence an individual's ability to function in society.

Advances in medical care are prolonging the lives of individuals who once may not have survived a chronic disease or severe injury. Yet, increased survival does not equate to restoration of function, and many individuals surviving life-threatening illnesses have long-term functional loss and disability. This has led to an increasing number of individuals receiving disability benefits and, in turn, has had a significant financial impact on society.[5] The increasing prevalence and financial issues are further compounded by poorly standardized disability-related terminology and evaluation procedures—all of which have raised serious problems for agencies determining and awarding disability benefits.[5]

In an effort to resolve some of the existing problems, US and international organizations have begun to examine terminology, evaluation procedures, and the relationship between disease presence and functional capacity. Over the last 5 to 6 decades, the consequences of disease have become known as "disablement."[5] Disablement frameworks have been developed to categorize or "organize information about the consequences of disease."[6(p5)]

DISABLEMENT FRAMEWORKS

Common disablement frameworks that have emerged include (1) the International Classification of Functioning, Disability, and Health (ICF),[7] developed by the WHO; (2) the Nagi framework,[5] developed by Saad Nagi; and (3) the National Center for Medical Rehabilitation Research (NCMRR) disability classification scheme.[8]

Nagi model - older model

International Classification of Functioning, Disability, and Health

The ICF, originally known as the International Classification of Impairments, Disabilities, and Handicaps (ICIDH), was endorsed by the 54th World Health Assembly and released in 2001. The operational definitions listed here have been endorsed by the WHO as part of the ICF[7(pp3,12-14)]:

Activity	Completion of a task or action by an individual
Participation	Involvement in a life situation
Impairment	A problem with body function (physiological or psychological) or structure (limb, organ) such as a deviation from or loss of what would be considered normal. Impairments may be directly related to the health condition or a result of another impairment (ie, postural abnormalities due to muscle imbalance)
	Impairments can be considered permanent or temporary; progressive, regressive, or static; intermittent or continuous; slight or severe; fluctuating
Activity limitations	Difficulties that might be encountered by an individual who is attempting to complete a <u>task</u> or carry out an activity
Participation restrictions	Problems an individual might face while involved in <u>life situations</u>
Functioning	Encompasses bodily functions, activities, and participation
Disability	Encompasses impairments, activity limitations, and participation restrictions.

One aim of the ICF is to provide a common language for describing functional status and disability according to health and health-related states.[7] The ICF blends anatomical and physiological impairments, physical functioning (including individual and societal roles), and contextual factors (those factors related to the surroundings or setting). This is accomplished by categorizing information about an individual's health condition into 2 distinct but related parts: (1) Functioning and Disability and (2) Contextual Factors[7] (Figure 1-1). Part 1, Functioning and Disability, is further divided into 2 components: (1) Body Functions and Structures and (2) Activities and Participation. Part 2,

things happening in the world that affects function(i.e. assistive devices)

things you can't change

	Part 1: Functioning and Disability		Part 2: Contextual Factors	
Components	Body Functions and Structures	Activities and Participation	Environmental Factors	Personal Factors
Domains	Body functions Body structures	Life areas (tasks, actions)	External influences on functioning and disability	Internal influences on functioning and disability
Constructs *Conceptual Components*	Change in body functions (physiological) Change in body structures (anatomical)	Capacity -- Executing tasks in a standard environment Performance -- Executing tasks in the current environment	Facilitating or hindering impact of features (attributes) of the physical, social, and attitudinal world	Impact of attributes of the person
Positive aspect	Functional and structural integrity	Activities Participation	Facilitators	Not applicable
	Functioning			
Negative aspect	Impairment *Change from norm*	Activity limitation Participation restriction	Barriers/hindrances	Not applicable
	Disability			

Figure 1-1. The International Classification of Functioning, Disability, and Health (ICF) from the World Health Organization. (Reprinted with permission from the World Health Organization [WHO]).

Contextual Factors, is composed of (1) Environmental Factors and (2) Personal Factors.

Under the "Body Functions and Structures" component of the framework, physiological and anatomical functions and structures are listed. Using this framework, the health care provider examines the individual and determines if deviations from "normal" exist. This allows for the identification of body systems that are uninvolved (or intact [positive aspects]) and involved (or impaired [negative aspects]).[9,10] For the next component, "Activities and Participation," activities are defined as "the execution of a task or action."[7(p10)] These are isolated tasks or functional activities such as brushing teeth, combing hair, and dressing. Participation is defined as "involvement in life situations."[9(p4)] Participation includes performance of socially constructed activities such as work, school, or community involvement. Under the Activities and Participation component, the ICF provides a set of functional activities and tasks (Figure 1-2). Using this sys-

tem, the examiner identifies tasks and life situations in which the individual can perform (positive aspects of the health condition) as well as those in which the individual *cannot* perform (negative aspects of the health condition). The online version of the ICF can be found at http://apps.who.int/classifications/icfbrowser/.

According to the WHO,[7] there can be difficulty differentiating between activities and participation. In looking back to the proposed definitions, an *activity* is simply a task or action carried out by an individual, whereas *participation* is involvement in a life situation. The WHO has suggested ways that health care practitioners can operationally define or differentiate between activities and participation. These include (1) to designate some functional skills as activities and some as participation (no overlap); (2) to designate some functional skills as activities and some as participation (with overlap); (3) to name detailed skills as activities and broad skills as participation; or (4) to call all skills

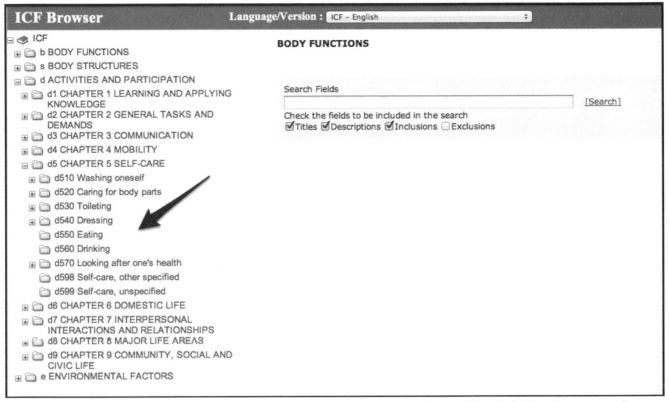

Figure 1-2. Screenshot of the International Classification of Functioning, Disability, and Health (ICF) online version showing a sample of tasks and activities found in the Activities and Participation component.

"activities and participation," not differentiating between the two.[7]

Contextual factors include environmental and personal factors that influence societal participation, either positively or negatively. Environmental factors are external factors, either immediate or global, that affect the individual as he or she interacts with society. More specifically, they "make up the physical, social and attitudinal environment in which people live and conduct their lives."[7(p16)] Things that facilitate interaction with the environment (ie, wheelchair ramps) are considered "positive aspects," whereas things that hinder interaction, or prevent the individual from participating in the environment, are known as "negative aspects." Examples include others' opinions or attitudes as well as physical barriers such as curbs and stairs. Personal factors are factors that are unique to the individual, such as age, race, gender, comorbidities, fitness level, or personal attributes.

The ICF is one classification system under the World Health Organization Family of International Classifications, or WHO-FIC.[4] The primary purpose of the WHO-FIC is to provide a uniform, standard language to describe health, disease, function, disability, and interventions. Other WHO-FIC classification systems are the International Statistical Classification of Diseases and Related Health Problems, Tenth Revision (ICD-10), which is a classification system for medical diagnoses and diseases, and the International Classification of Health Interventions (ICHI), a classification of curative and preventive health interventions.[11] The 3 classifications are designed to complement one another. At the time of this publication, the US health care system was using a prior version of the ICD, the ICD Ninth Revision, or ICD-9. There are plans to transition to the ICD-10 at some time in the future. The WHO-FIC is recommended for use by and is provided to governments, health care providers, consumers, and researchers worldwide.[4] Standard classification systems and language facilitate the storage, retrieval, and comparison of disease-related data in health care systems throughout the world.[4]

The Nagi Disablement Framework

Another disablement framework, the Nagi framework, was developed in the 1960s by sociologist Saad Nagi in response to the vast number of definitions for disability that existed, inconsistency in disability assessment, and disparity over awarding disability benefits based solely on impairments.[6] The Nagi framework provided the following terms and definitions as a conceptual framework linking pathology to disability (Figure 1-3):

- *Active pathology* — usually diseases (diabetes)
- *Impairment* — change from normal
- *Functional limitation* — activity/task you can't do
- *Disability*

In this framework, *active pathology* is defined as the interruption or interference with the body's normal processes and simultaneous body efforts to heal itself or regain

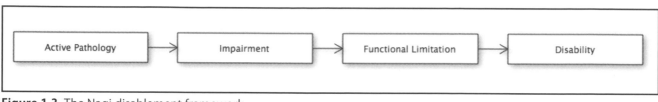

Figure 1-3. The Nagi disablement framework.

a normal state. A pathology can result from a variety of causes, including trauma and degenerative changes.[5] The pathology is often referred to as the disease itself; occurs at the cellular, tissue, or organ level; and is often the patient's medical diagnosis.[12] Medical management and physician interventions are often directed at reducing the active pathology. Examples of active pathologies include osteoporosis, Parkinson disease, and fracture.

Impairment is a loss or abnormality of an anatomical, physiological, mental, or emotional nature.[5] Impairments are deviations from normal occurring at the cellular, tissue, organ, or system level. Nagi[5] described 3 types of impairments. The first is the disease process itself because the disease represents a deviation from normal anatomy or physiology. The second type of impairment is the *result* of the pathology. These impairments comprise the signs and/or symptoms of the active pathology, or the problems remaining once the pathology has been resolved. The third type of impairment is one not caused by the pathology but, instead, is a result of a congenital problem, such as a postural abnormality like scoliosis or clubfoot. In physical therapy, the 2 latter types are given the most consideration. Besides postural abnormalities, impairments often encountered in physical therapy practice include decreased range of motion or joint immobility, muscle weakness, faulty balance, and impaired sensation.

A *functional limitation* refers to an abnormality or limitation in an individual's ability to carry out a meaningful action, task, and/or activity in an efficient, competent, reasonably expected manner.[5,12] In the Nagi framework, functional limitations are experienced at the "organism" level, or as the individual functions "as a whole."[5] Functional limitations are specific to the individual and are based on the demands and activities of his or her lifestyle. This is a task or activity the individual *could* do prior to the onset of the pathology. For example, following an elbow fracture, a 25-year-old man is limited in elbow flexion in the dominant extremity and cannot feed himself. In this example, the active pathology is the fracture, the impairment is decreased elbow range of motion, and the functional limitation is self-feeding with the dominant extremity.

Impairments often cause or contribute to functional limitations. In the previous example, the range of motion impairment is causing the functional limitation. Also, an individual with limited hip range of motion (impairment) might have difficulty sitting and standing from a chair or have difficulty donning pants (functional limitations) because of the hip immobility. In addition, a patient with decreased quadriceps strength (impairment) might have difficulty ascending and descending stairs (functional limitations) because of weakness.

However, functional limitations are not solely dependent on the type, number, *or* severity of the impairments.

Rather, the combination of the impairment and an individual's normal activities, tasks, roles, and responsibilities will determine the functional limitation(s). Consider the following examples. There are two 65-year-old women who have degenerative joint disease in both hips. Both have pain, decreased hip joint range of motion, decreased strength, and decreased gait velocity. Patient 1 lives in a 2-story house, so for her a functional limitation is ascending and descending stairs. Patient 2 lives in a single-level home but enjoys playing on the floor with her grandchildren. For patient 2, rising and lowering to the floor are functional limitations. As you can see, these women have similar impairments but different functional limitations because of their lifestyles.

Disability, the fourth aspect of the Nagi framework, is the inability or limitation in performing socially defined roles and/or tasks that would normally be expected of an individual of similar gender or age within a given culture and/or environment.[5] These roles and tasks are organized by life activities and often include (1) self-care, (2) home management, (3) work, (4) community activities, and (5) leisure activities.[12] Let us look at 2 more patients. Patient 1 is a 52-year-old male accountant who spends the majority of his day at his computer. Patient 2 is a 45-year-old mechanic who works with his arms elevated overhead 75% of the day. Both patients have been diagnosed with shoulder impingement syndrome (active pathology) and have limited shoulder range of motion (impairment). Both have difficulty reaching overhead because of pain (functional limitation). However, patient 1 is able to perform normal work duties, but patient 2 is not able to work because of his inability to reach overhead without pain. For patient 1, the result of the impairment is less profound. You can see from this example that individuals with similar impairments and functional limitations might have differing degrees of disability. The patient working as a mechanic could be considered "temporarily disabled" in his ability to work (a role that is socially expected of him), whereas the accountant continues to perform the role that is normally expected of him and would not be considered to have a disability in work.

There is often an overlap between an individual's functional limitations and his or her disabilities. The reason is that a specific activity or task carried out by an individual may also be a socially defined role or responsibility. Consider the individual with the elbow fracture. Some would say that self-feeding is both a functional limitation and a socially expected activity for someone of his age and, therefore, his inability to feed himself would also be a disability.

In many cases, functional limitations result in compensatory behaviors. When a patient cannot perform a common task in the normal manner, he or she may identify another way to do it. Many times, the role of the physical therapist (PT) is to assist the patient or family in identifying compensatory strategies to perform normal functional tasks. In considering the case of the patient with an elbow fracture, his compensatory strategy might be eating with his nondominant extremity. According to the Nagi framework,[5] disability results when the patient is *unable* to return to what would normally be expected. When the patient identifies a compensatory strategy that is effective, efficient, and allows return to his or her normal socially identified role, then the patient would not be considered "disabled."

Another consideration when correlating functional limitations and disability are comorbidities, or prior medical conditions that complicate the patient's current problem. If the patient with the elbow fracture had previously had a stroke with resultant paralysis of the nondominant extremity, now the functional limitation—self-feeding—is a larger issue because the patient cannot use the uninvolved extremity. The patient will remain disabled in self-feeding until the he regains normal range of motion or finds an efficient, effective way to eat.

Nagi[5] provided 3 additional factors that influence an individual's perception of his or her disability. These include (1) the individual's situation and his or her reactions to the situation; (2) the situation and reactions of others, such as family, friends, associates, and coworkers; and (3) the presence of environmental barriers.[5] These additional factors are paralleled in the ICF (part 2, Contextual Factors) that includes global and immediate environmental factors as well as personal factors.

As you can see, relating disability concepts is complex and can be confusing. Let us summarize a few disablement concepts according to Nagi using a final example.

Point #1: There is overlap between functional limitation and disability.

A 24-year-old man is involved in a motor vehicle accident and sustains an L2-L3 incomplete spinal cord injury. He has weakness in many of his major lower extremity muscles causing knee and ankle instability during gait. He ambulates 25 feet on level surfaces with an assistive device and assistance from the PT.

> *Active pathology:* Incomplete L2-L3 spinal cord injury
>
> *Impairment:* Decreased muscle strength
>
> *Functional limitation:* Impaired mobility and gait
>
> *Disability:* Impaired mobility and gait. For a healthy 24-year-old man, independent, normal ambulation for unlimited distances is an expectation.

Point #2: Compensatory strategies, including the use of assistive devices, can allow people to overcome functional limitations and return to normal activities.

The patient learns to ambulate with ankle-foot orthoses and Lofstrand crutches. With the assistive devices, he can ambulate unlimited distances independently without fatiguing. Without the assistive devices, he requires assistance, his gait is inefficient, and he fatigues quickly.

Point #3: Comorbidities influence the way people adapt to their functional limitations and may increase the likelihood of resulting disability.

The patient later develops a chronic lung condition and has difficulty breathing during activities that cause exertion. He can walk only short distances with the assistive devices becasue of poor endurance and he requires a wheelchair for longer distances.

The National Center for Medical Rehabilitation Research Classification Scheme for Disability Terminology

The National Center for Medical Rehabilitation Research (NCMRR) is a branch of the National Institute of Child Health and Human Development of the National Institutes of Health (NIH). In the early 1990s, Congress directed the NIH to establish a special committee to provide guidance to the NCMRR. This special committee, the National Advisory Board on Medical Rehabilitation Research (NABMRR), provided direction for rehabilitation research initiatives to the NCMRR. The goal was for the Advisory Board to assist the NIH in extending the same excellence to rehabilitation science research that was extended to biological science research. The hope was to improve research related to improving function and enhancing quality of life for people with disabilities.[8]

Acknowledging previously developed disablement frameworks, the NABMRR indicated that none of them suited their intent to describe the role of rehabilitation in improving function and quality of life. Consequently, the NABMRR identified 5 domains relevant to rehabilitation, pathophysiology, impairment, functional limitation, disability, and societal limitation.[8] Definitions provided for these domains are as follows[8(pp5,23-25)]:

Pathophysiology	An interruption of, or interference with normal physiological and developmental processes or structures; occurs at the cellular or tissue level
Impairment	A loss or abnormality of cognitive, emotional, physiological, or anatomical structure or function; occurs in the organ, or organ system
Functional Limitation	Restriction or lack of ability to perform the task designated to perform; abnormal function of an organism
Disability	Inability or limitation in performance of tasks, activities, and roles at levels typically expected within a given social context; occurs at the level of the individual
Societal Limitation	Restriction due to social policy or barriers, physical or attitudinal, limiting the fulfillment of roles or denying access to services and

opportunities associated with full societal participation (ie, vocation, housing, health care, etc); occurs at the societal level, or how the individual functions within society

In putting forth this framework, the NABMRR suggested a "Research Plan" in which these domains would serve as "five overlapping domains of research that are relevant to studying disability."[8(p9)]

In summary, the WHO, Nagi, and NCMRR have provided frameworks, or conceptual models, for defining disability terminology and examining the relationship between disease, impairments, limitations in function, and disability. In addition, these frameworks provide a mechanism for allowing clinicians and researchers to be aware of the impact of disease on an individual's day-to-day life and overall function within society. Consideration of a disablement model when working with patients helps health care providers to realize more complex, psychosocial issues that patients face because of the health condition, disease, or injury.

DISABLEMENT AND PHYSICAL THERAPY

Individuals in need of physical therapy services often have a disease or injury with resulting impairments. It is our responsibility to understand how these impairments affect their functional, day-to-day activities—in a variety of settings and situations. Disablement models have been a topic in physical therapy literature for the last 2 to 3 decades, and the discussion regarding the disablement framework best suited for use in physical therapy practice has shifted back and forth between the WHO model and the Nagi model. In 1989, Jette[13] put forth the idea of PTs using a disablement framework, primarily for patient diagnosis and classification. He explained how the ICIDH (now called the ICF) provided a structure for classifying information gathered during a physical therapy examination. In using the model, the PT not only documented the patient's medical diagnosis but also provided the "impairment diagnosis," and the "handicap diagnosis."[13(p88)] Outlining the different diagnoses allowed for the provision of information on the consequences of disease, which tends to be a primary focus of physical therapy intervention.[13]

In 1991, Guccione[14] reported limitations in using the ICIDH in physical therapy and recommended using the Nagi framework. In supporting the Nagi framework, he provided reasons that it was more useful than the ICIDH and identified ways that the Nagi model could be modified to further meet the needs of PTs. Guccione's expanded version of Nagi's framework was adopted for use in the second edition of the *Guide to Physical Therapist Practice* to serve as a framework for physical therapy practice and diagnosis.[12]

In 1994, Verbrugge and Jette[15] discussed disablement as a "process" that is influenced by nonmedical factors such as social, environmental, and psychological factors. They identified the influences of (1) risk factors, or predisposing factors that may prompt or endure disablement; (2) interventions, such as physical therapy, used to reduce disability; and (3) intrinsic and external factors that exacerbate disability.[15] Keeping with the Nagi framework as the main pathway from pathology to disability, yet realizing facilitating and inhibiting factors to the disablement process, Verbrugge and Jette[15] proposed an alternate sociomedical model influenced by the environmental demands and individual capabilities.

In 2006, Jette[16] identified a need for a common language in physical therapy clinical practice and research. In this article, traditional frameworks were discussed and the author concluded that the ICF held great promise to "provide the rehabilitation disciplines with a universal language with which to discuss disability."[16(p733)] In July 2008, the American Physical Therapy Association House of Delegates voted to endorse the ICF, which includes using ICF language in all future publications, documents, and communications.[17]

Over the last 5 to 6 years, there has been an increase in ICF integration in physical therapy publications. These publications have focused on various uses of the ICF in clinical practice.[18] Authors have identified ways commonly used outcome questionnaires reflect ICF concepts, thus helping clinicians in the selection of appropriate measures to examine patient impairment and function. Authors have also used the ICF as a framework for developing and writing clinical guidelines and for categorizing health effects after injuries. The use of the ICF as an evaluation tool is still under investigation.[19]

In using the ICF evaluation scheme, ICF items are scored on a scale of 0 (no difficulty) to 4 (complete difficulty).[9] Consideration is also given to the environmental factors and whether they act as a barrier or facilitator.[19] Items may also be scored as "not specified" or "not applicable."[9] PTs have traditionally not used this scale as part of their patient examination, but its validity and reliability are under investigation.[19]

Another clinical application of the ICF has been through the core sets. The ICF is very comprehensive and includes many items that may not be appropriate for each patient encountered in daily practice.[20] In fact, there may be only a small percentage, or "core set," of items in the ICF that are appropriate for a patient's diagnosis or injury. Core sets include body structures and functions, activities and participation, and environmental factors that are specific to a particular disease or injury and can be used to aid in patient evaluation at any point along the disease process or continuum of care. The ICF Research Branch and the WHO have developed a rigorous scientific process on developing core sets.[20] There are core sets for MS, spinal cord injury, traumatic brain injury, chronic obstructive pulmonary disease, osteoporosis, osteoarthritis, rheumatoid arthritis, and hand conditions, along with many others that would be relevant to physical therapy.[20]

participation. Documentation should describe the effects of treatment not only on impairments but also on function.

DISABLEMENT AND DOCUMENTATION

Documentation, otherwise known as medical record keeping, has been defined as "any entry into the patient-client record, such as a(n) consultation reports, initial examination reports, progress notes, flow sheets, checklists, reexamination reports, or summations of care that identifies the care or service provided."[12(p703)] Redgate and Foto[21] indicated that complete documentation also includes the physician prescription(s) and certification(s), communication with other care providers, copies of exercise programs or patient instructions, as well as any other care providers' notes or comments that support the interventions provided.

As you have read, there is a need in physical therapy for a common language, or consistency in terminology. One way to accomplish this from a clinical perspective is through consistency in our documentation, because our "notes" are the sole record of the episode of care provided to each patient or client. Disablement frameworks provide terms and concepts that can be integrated into our documentation to improve consistency in the language used in documentation.

Disablement concepts can be integrated into the initial examination. The physical therapy examination will detect the individual's impairments. These are often limitations in range of motion, strength, balance, etc; however, the examination must go beyond the impairment level to identify the consequences of disease and see how the patient's ability to function has been compromised. This includes documenting the patient's ability or inability to perform meaningful activities or tasks, such as hygiene or dressing, and participate in normal life situations, such as work- or school-related functions. It is also important for the PT to describe how the impairment(s) are impacting or causing the functional deficit(s). In traditional physical therapy documentation formats, however, the relationship(s) between impairment and function are often omitted or implied. Clinicians have also assumed that documented impairments indicate functional problems. This has resulted in documentation that provides an unclear or inadequate picture of the patient. The reader is often left to draw his or her own conclusions as to how the impairments are influencing function.

Integrating disablement terminology in documentation can also be done by way of describing how the interventions have influenced impairment, function, and participation. The physical therapy interventions are often aimed at reducing the individual's impairments. For example, we teach patients to perform range of motion and strengthening exercises. In doing these exercises, we hope to not only reduce impairments but to also improve function and

SUMMARY

Disablement is becoming an increasingly more important aspect of the health care system in which we function. PTs need consistency across the profession, and one way to achieve that is to integrate disablement terms and concepts. Several ways to integrate disablement concepts are outlined in this section (Figure 1-4) and serve as the foundation of this textbook. As you will read in subsequent chapters, documentation serves many purposes and there are many styles and formats for physical therapy records. Regardless of the style that you are using, your documentation should use consistent disablement terminology.

APPLICATION EXERCISE

1. Determine whether the following is (are) pathology (P), impairment (I), activity limitation (AL), or participation restriction (PR) according to the ICF.

    a. _I_ Elbow flexion contracture

    b. _?_ Right hip osteoarthritis

    c. _PR_ A 48-year-old man requires a wheelchair for community mobility and can self-propel 200 feet on level surfaces prior to fatigue

    d. _AL_ Difficulty opening a heavy door

    e. _PR_ A patient with impaired mobility is unable to go to the grocery store because of lack of a wheelchair ramp at the grocery store entrance

    f. _I_ Decreased shoulder range of motion

    g. _P_ Emphysema

    h. _P_ Congenital hip dysplasia

    i. _AL_ A 55-year-old man is unable to open a jar because of weakness following a cerebrovascular accident

    j. _PR_ A 15-year-old girl with spastic quadriplegia is unable to participate in physical education class with her peers

2. Determine whether the following is (are) pathology (P), impairment (I), functional limitation (FL), or disability (D) according to the Nagi framework.

    a. _P_ Right transtibial amputation

    b. _I_ Knee flexion contracture

    c. _FL_ A 52-year-old man requires minimal assist for household ambulation

    d. _D_ A patient with impaired mobility is unable to leave his house because of lack of a wheelchair ramp at the house entrance

    e. _I_ Poor balance

Figure 1-4. Ways to integrate disablement concepts into physical therapy documentation.

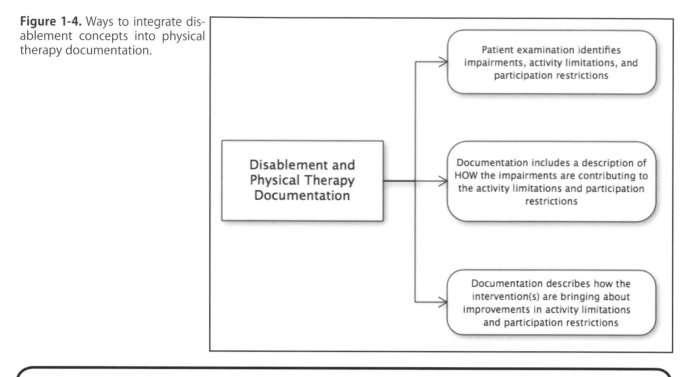

REVIEW QUESTIONS

1. In your own words, define disablement. Give an example of how a person can be disabled according to the definition you provided. the results of a disease - someone who has an amputated food due to uncontrolled Diabetes

2. How is the "medical model" of health different from the "biopsychosocial model" of health?
   medical model - free of disease
   biopsychosocial model - complete physical, mental, & social well-being

3. List reasons for the development of disablement frameworks.

4. List the major disablement frameworks.

5. Complete the table here using terminology from the ICF, the Nagi framework, and NCMRR using the following terms: pathology or pathophysiology, impairment, functional limitation, disability, activity limitation, participation restriction, and societal limitation.

	ICF	Nagi	NCMRR
A patient's medical diagnosis			
Loss or abnormality of an individual's anatomy or physiology			
Difficulties that are encountered when an individual attempts to complete a task			
The inability to carry out a normal activity because of a problem with the anatomy or physiology			

Problems an individual faces while involved in life situations			
Encompasses impairments and limitations in abilities to carry out socially acceptable tasks			
Unable to carry out a task that would be socially appropriate for an individual			

6. What is the difference between
    a. Activity limitation and participation restriction?
    b. Environmental and personal factors?
    c. Positive and negative aspects of disease according to the ICF?
    d. Functional limitation and disability?

7. How are impairments and functional limitations related?

8. How are impairments, functional limitations, and disability related?

9. What is the WHO-FIC? What makes up the WHO-FIC? Why is it recommended?

10. What disablement frameworks have been proposed for use in physical therapy?

11. Which disablement framework was most recently adopted for use by the American Physical Therapy Association House of Delegates?

12. The Nagi framework implies that pathology leads to impairment. Do you think impairment can lead to pathology? Why or why not? If so, give an example.

13. What is a core set? How can they be used in physical therapy?

14. How should disablement be reflected in documentation?

15. Research the core set for a condition commonly treated by PTs. How is it laid out? How can it be useful in practice?

f. __I__ Poor endurance

g. __D__ A 35-year-old man is unable to work on an assembly line in a meat packing plant because of a shoulder injury

h. __P__ Cerebral palsy

i. __FL__ A 65-year-old woman with rheumatoid arthritis uses a button hook to dress because of hand weakness and deformity

j. __FL__ A 20-year-old man uses a sliding board and moderate assistance to transfer from bed to wheelchair following a spinal cord injury

3. Read the following scenarios and determine the following:

- pathology
- activity limitation(s)
- participation restriction(s)
- environmental factors/facilitator(s)
- environmental factors/barrier(s)
- *possible* personal factors that could potentially influence the situation

a. You are working with a 10-year-old girl in the school system. Her medical diagnosis is spastic diplegia. You have been working on ambulating up and down the stairs (which she can perform with minimal assist of 1 and a quad cane and handrail) and increasing the speed of her gait. At the present time, she leaves her classes early so that she can make it to the next one on time, and she uses the elevator rather than the stairs.

b. Your patient is a 35-year-old man who sustained a traumatic, closed head injury in a motorcycle accident. He is confused and disoriented, and he requires constant supervision for his safety. He can perform activities of daily living (ADL) with supervision and occasional verbal cues. He can walk and get in and out of bed with supervision. He can also ascend and descend stairs with supervision. He has not returned to work as a radiologic technician since his injury.

REFERENCES

1. Law M. *Evidence-Based Rehabilitation: A Guide to Practice.* Thorofare, NJ: SLACK Incorporated; 2002.
2. Wade DT, Halligan PW. Do biomedical models of illness make for good healthcare systems? *BMJ.* 2004;329(7479):1398-1401.
3. World Health Organization. WHO definition of health: Official Records of the World Health Organization: Preamble to the Constitution of the World Health Organization as adopted by the International Conference (New York, 19–22 June 1946) by the Representatives of the 61 states. http://www.who.int/about/definition/en/print.html. Accessed May 10, 2012.
4. World Health Organization. The WHO Family of International Classifications. http://www.who.int/classifications/en/. Accessed May 10, 2012.
5. Nagi S. Disability concepts revisited: implications for prevention. In: Pope AM, Tarlov AR, eds. *Disability in America: Toward a National Agenda for Prevention.* Washington, DC: National Academy Press; 1991:309-327.
6. Pope A, Tarlov A. *Disability in America: Toward a National Agenda for Prevention.* Washington, DC: National Academy Press; 1991.
7. World Health Organization. *International Classification of Functioning, Disability and Health: ICF.* Geneva, Switzerland: World Health Organization; 2001.
8. National Advisory Board on Medical Rehabilitation Research. *Research Plan for the National Center for Medical Rehabilitation Research.* Rockville, MD: National Institutes of Health; 1993. NIH publication 93-3509.
9. World Health Organization. ICF checklist. http://www.who.int/classifications/icf/training/icfchecklist.pdf. Accessed June 28, 2012.
10. World Health Organization. ICF classification hypertext version. http://apps.who.int/classifications/icfbrowser/. Accessed May 10, 2012.
11. World Health Organization. International Classification of Health Interventions. http://www.who.int/classifications/ichi/en/. Accessed May 10, 2012.
12. American Physical Therapy Association. *Guide to Physical Therapist Practice.* 2nd ed. Alexandria, VA: APTA; 2003.
13. Jette AM. Diagnosis and classification by physical therapists: a special communication. *Phys Ther.* 1989;69:87-89.
14. Guccione A. Physical therapy diagnosis and the relationship between impairments and function. *Phys Ther.* 1991;71(7):10-14.
15. Verbrugge LM, Jette AM. The disablement process. *Soc Sci Med.* 1994;38(1):1-14.
16. Jette AM. Toward a common language for function, disability, and health. *Phys Ther.* 2006;86(5):726-734.
17. American Physical Therapy Association. APTA endorses World Health Organization ICF model. http://www.apta.org/Media/Releases/APTA/2008/7/8/. Accessed May 10, 2012.
18. Escorpizo R, Bemis-Dougherty A, Davenport TE, Feliciano H, Vreeman DJ, Riddle DL. The ICF and physical therapy 10 years later. Presented at: Combined Sections Meeting of the American Physical Therapy Association; February 10, 2012; Chicago, IL.
19. Grill E, Gloor-Juzi T, Huber EO, Stucki G. Operationalization and reliability testing of ICF categories relevant for physiotherapists' interventions in the acute hospital. *J Rehabil Med.* 2011;43(2):162-173.
20. ICF Research Branch. ICF core set projects. http://www.icf-research-branch.org/icf-core-sets-projects-sp-1641021024398. Accessed May 10, 2012.
21. Redgate N, Foto M. Pay by the rules: avoid Medicare audits and reduce payment denials with a sound strategy and proper documentation. *Physical Therapy Products.* 2003;October/November:28-30.

Chapter 2

Reasons for Documenting in Physical Therapy

Mia L. Erickson, PT, EdD, CHT, ATC

CHAPTER OUTLINE

Record Patient/Client Management
Communicate With Others
Demonstrate Clinical Problem Solving
Support Reimbursement and Need for Services
Provide Proof That Care Is "Reasonable and Necessary" and "Medically Necessary"
Provide Proof of Skilled Care
Facilitate Administrative Duties
Serve as a Legal Record of Care

CHAPTER OBJECTIVES

Upon completion of this chapter, the reader will be able to:
1. List reasons for documenting in physical therapy.
2. List components of patient/client management that are included in documentation.
3. Explain how other providers use physical therapy documentation.
4. Explain how documentation demonstrates clinical problem solving.
5. Explain the physical therapist assistant's role in the clinical decision-making process.
6. Examine the relationship between reimbursement and documentation.
7. Describe reasonable and necessary criteria and skilled care.
8. Differentiate between skilled care and maintenance therapy.
9. List situations when maintenance therapy can be considered skilled care.
10. Describe how documentation can be used in legal matters.

Erickson ML, Utzman RR, McKnight R. *Physical Therapy Documentation: From Examination to Outcome, Second Edition* (pp 13-20).
© 2014 SLACK Incorporated.

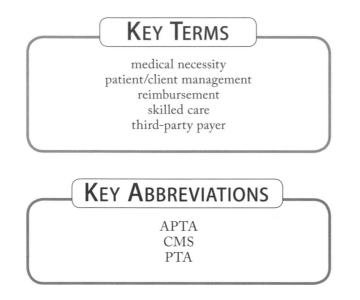

KEY TERMS

medical necessity
patient/client management
reimbursement
skilled care
third-party payer

KEY ABBREVIATIONS

APTA
CMS
PTA

RECORD PATIENT/CLIENT MANAGEMENT

One of the primary reasons for documenting in physical therapy is to maintain a record of how we manage a patient/client (Figure 2-1).[1] In documenting patient/client management, the PT creates and provides evidence of the episode of care that begins with the physical therapy referral (unless the patient accesses physical therapy through direct access) and concludes with the discharge summary, or summary of

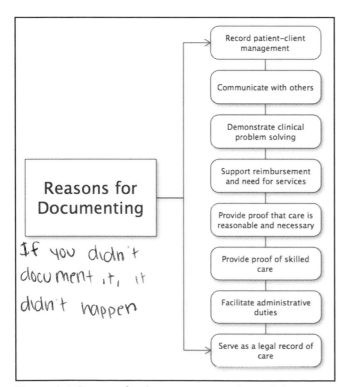

Figure 2-1. Reasons for documenting in physical therapy.

the final outcome. The documentation includes all relevant patient data, the PT's assessment of the patient's condition, all interventions provided, and other information that is provided in later chapters. The law requires health care providers to maintain a record of health care provided to patients. Accurate documentation is also an ethical responsibility, as outlined in the *Code of Ethics for the Physical Therapist*.[2]

COMMUNICATE WITH OTHERS

Records of patient data and care provided are important to other individuals involved in the patient's management, and these records serve as a useful means of communication. Other health care providers including physicians, nurses, occupational and speech therapists, and case managers are often interested in a patient's status, and these individuals often need to refer to the physical therapy documentation. For example, in an inpatient hospital setting, a physician might be interested in how safely and independently a patient can ambulate when deciding whether to send the patient home. Nurses might be interested in a patient's ability to transfer in and out of bed and case managers often need to identify equipment needs or return-to-work status. Therefore, documenting patient data serves as a useful tool for facilitating communication across disciplines.

In addition to communication with nonphysical therapy providers, documentation serves as a reference for individuals who work with your patients in your absence. It is important that the PT's documentation provides accurate and clear information for the individual assuming the care of the patient. Clearly written notes help those treating provide appropriate and consistent care much more efficiently. Transfer of physical therapy services from one setting to another (eg, acute care to home health) is also quite common, and well-written notes can facilitate continuity of care across settings. Transfer of care can also happen between 2 PTs and between PTs and physical therapist assistants (PTAs).

A PTA assuming the care of the patient relies on the PT's documentation to provide information and direction. The PT's documentation informs the PTA regarding the patient's diagnosis, prognosis, and status, so he or she knows what to expect and how to prepare for seeing the patient the first time. This might include things such as level of assist needed for transfers and assistive device used during gait. The PT's documentation also alerts the PTA to any precautions or restrictions such as weight-bearing status, allergies, or special indications or contraindications for treatment. The PTA uses the PT's documentation and plan of care to provide the correct intervention(s) and progression.[3]

DEMONSTRATE CLINICAL PROBLEM SOLVING

At each patient encounter, PTs use clinical problem-solving skills and clinical judgment to determine how to manage each patient. Physical therapy documentation reflects and summarizes the clinician's problem solving and judgment.[4–6] The medical record tells a story of the patient's physical therapy encounter. Any individual who does not know the patient should be able to read the physical therapy documentation and identify the patient's impairments and functional problems as well as steps taken to specifically address each one. Documentation that demonstrates clinical problem solving also improves the provider's credibility with third-party payers.[7]

Any individual who provides aspects of patient/client management is responsible for ensuring the patient's record reflects clinical problem solving. Recall from Chapter 1, when integrating disablement into documentation, the PT clearly documents impairments, activity limitations, and participation restrictions using appropriate, objective tests and measures. In addition, the PT describes, in a summary, how the impairments are limiting the patient's functional abilities. This can help support the clinician's clinical problem solving.

Another way to integrate clinical problem solving is to describe the adequacy of the interventions provided. This was also mentioned in Chapter 1. Both the PT and PTA describe how a specific intervention is bringing about change in an impairment, activity limitation, or participation restriction. This strategy can further demonstrate the clinical problem-solving process.

Take a look at the following list of specific ways the PT and PTA can demonstrate clinical problem solving in the clinical documentation.

During the examination:
- The PT collects data during the initial examination and draws the reader's attention to the problem areas (eg, impairments, activity limitations, and participation restrictions) in the summary and plan of care. The PT develops a plan that includes specific interventions aimed at addressing the identified patient problems. For example, a patient with

poor endurance is treated with a program that includes cardiovascular activities aimed at building endurance, and a patient with poor balance has a home exercise program that provides specific balance activities.

At subsequent therapy sessions:
- The PT and PTA collect pertinent subjective and objective data at subsequent therapy sessions and record them in interim notes. Subjective data collected during this phase include (1) asking the patient about his or her response to a previous treatment, (2) inquiring about adherence with an exercise program, or (3) asking the patient if the treatment has improved function. Objective data include relevant tests and measures that are consistent with those from the initial examination. Therapists compare subjective remarks and results of tests and measures between current and prior visits. PTs and PTAs explicitly state changes in patient status in the documentation and bring them to the reader's attention. For example, document, "The patient's range of motion for the left shoulder improved from 90 to 120 degrees in 1 week" or "The patient ambulated 150' today with minimal assist of 1 to advance the left lower extremity compared to 50' with moderate assist of 2, 1 week ago."
- The PT and PTA adjust the intervention when the patient's status changes, either positively or negatively. When changes are significant, the PT adjusts the plan of care.
- The PT and PTA document changes brought about by the intervention. For example, you have been working with a patient following a total knee arthroplasty. The patient has been limited in his ability to don his shoes and sit comfortably in a chair because of limited knee flexion. After 2 weeks of exercise, the patient's knee range of motion has improved 25 degrees. He is now able to sit more comfortably in a chair and don his shoes without assistance. The PT provides information regarding the improved impairment (range of motion) and the improved function (sitting and donning shoes), then provides a statement describing how the interventions have helped in the improvement (eg, "Range of motion exercises have helped in increasing knee flexion and now patient is able to sit more comfortably and don shoes independently").

Describing the clinical problem-solving process is an important aspect of documentation. Ongoing documentation of subjective remarks and objective findings tells the story of the patient's response to treatment. Consistency between the initial, interim, and discharge documentation makes it easier for a reader to identify and follow the clinical problem-solving process. In addition, consistency between initial and subsequent documentation makes it easier for the clinician(s) to identify progress or a lack thereof. Finally, comparing current data to that gathered during the initial examination allows the PT to easily update goals and interventions as needed.

SUPPORT REIMBURSEMENT AND NEED FOR SERVICES

In the 1960s, medical records existed to (1) provide a legal record of care, (2) facilitate communication among health care providers, and (3) serve as a source of information for clinical research.[8] In the 1970s, documentation became a reimbursement requirement by government agencies such as Medicare and Medicaid. Medicare began requiring rehabilitation facilities not only to maintain documentation but also to submit records to be reviewed by Medicare auditors. Auditors reviewed documentation to determine if physical therapy services provided to Medicare beneficiaries met requirements for reimbursement.[8]

Today, documentation is a requirement for all third-party payers to support reimbursement. Adequate documentation serves as a record of what was billed on a particular date of service and allows payers to verify treatment provided to a beneficiary. It is important to point out that, in the current health care system, third-party payers review and dissect physical therapy documentation more than ever. Many payers continue to conduct audits to determine if the documentation meets reimbursement requirements and supports payment for physical therapy services. Consider the following example.

You are working in a skilled nursing facility and you receive a phone call from a government agency that some of your billing practices have triggered an external audit. They are asking that you submit documentation from 15 patient charts for dates of service January 1 through June 30 from the previous year. The plan is for the agency to review the documentation and determine if it supports payment you received for these patients. If documentation DOES NOT support services billed, then the facility where you are working must pay back the money already reimbursed.

Audits can be devastating for facilities, managers, and therapists. They can also be financially draining. You can see from this example the importance of adequate documentation that supports what was billed in the event of an audit.

In addition to justifying interventions billed, especially in the event of an audit, documentation helps support the need for further physical therapy services. Consider this example.

You are a PT working in a small, outpatient private practice. For the last 6 weeks, you have been working with a 35-year-old man who was recently involved in a motorcycle accident. In the accident, he sustained a mild concussion and multiple left lower extremity fractures. Initially, he was unable to bear weight through the extremity and required a wheelchair for mobility. He had significant loss in range of motion and strength. He was unable to perform independent self-care, normal

home and community mobility including ambulation, or his usual work activities. Since the initial visit, he has been making excellent progress and is now able to walk using one crutch, weight bearing as tolerated, and he has resumed most of his normal ADL. After seeing him for 14 visits, it is brought to your attention that his insurance requires authorization for visits occurring after the initial 15. In order to have additional therapy services approved, you must submit adequate documentation showing evidence of (1) patient progress and (2) justification for continuing treatment.

Continuation of physical therapy benefits for this patient is based largely on how well you have objectively documented his improvement and how well you can justify that additional services are necessary for his condition.

As a therapist, it is difficult to stay abreast of documentation requirements for reimbursement, especially when you work with a diverse payer mix. Documentation requirements can also be somewhat elusive or vague. They can be difficult to find, interpret, and translate into clinical practice. The American Physical Therapy Association (APTA) provides guidelines for physical therapy documentation.[9,10] The Centers for Medicare & Medicaid Services (CMS) has also provided documentation requirements for those working with Medicare beneficiaries.[11] These resources can help physical therapy providers keep patient records that are appropriate for securing reimbursement or additional services and support services provided in the event of an audit.

PROVIDE PROOF THAT CARE IS "REASONABLE AND NECESSARY" AND "MEDICALLY NECESSARY"

Clinical documentation serves to justify that care provided to patients is reasonable and necessary. The phrase "reasonable and necessary" originated from language describing benefits covered under the Medicare system. In our clinical documentation, however, it is often difficult to articulate *how* services are reasonable and necessary. Nevertheless, it is expected to be an integral part of documentation in the event of an audit or when requesting additional services, especially for Medicare beneficiaries. In 2006, CMS published conditions that should be met in order for services to be considered reasonable and necessary in the outpatient therapy setting[11]:

- The services shall be considered under accepted standards of medical practice to be a specific and effective treatment for the patient's condition.

- The services provided to the patient are at a level of complexity and sophistication that can be provided only by a therapist or assistant, under appropriate supervision (see skilled care in next section).

- The condition of the patient is such that services can safely and effectively be provided only by a therapist or assistant, under appropriate supervision. While the patient's medical condition is an important factor in considering whether services are skilled, a beneficiary's diagnosis or prognosis should never be the sole factor in deciding that a service is or is not skilled.

- An expectation exists that the patient's condition will improve significantly in a reasonable (and generally predictable) period of time, or the services must be necessary for the establishment of a safe and effective maintenance program required in connection with a specific disease state. In the case of a progressive degenerative disease, service may be necessary to determine the need for assistive or adaptive equipment and/or to establish a program to maximize patient function.

- The amount, frequency, and duration of the services must be reasonable under accepted standards of practice in the local area or according to state or national therapy associations.

These conditions are used for general purposes but, since their implementation, CMS has provided more specific criteria for various physical therapy settings.[12–15] Other third-party payers besides Medicare may also use these conditions. It is the therapist's responsibility to stay abreast of conditions set forth by payers for what is considered reasonable and necessary.

A similar phrase used in practice is "medical necessity," or "medically necessary." There is no single well-accepted definition for medical necessity and many third-party payers provide their own definition. In general, medically necessary services are services or supplies that are needed for the diagnosis or treatment of a medical condition and meet accepted standards of medical practice.[16] Many people use the phrase "reasonable and necessary" and "medically necessary" interchangeably. When comparing the conditions of reasonable and necessary (listed above) and the definition of medical necessity, it seems that medical necessity is only one aspect of the reasonable and necessary criteria. Therapists should be familiar with all the reasonable and necessary criteria in addition to what is meant by medical necessary.

Physical therapists determine whether an intervention is reasonable and necessary based on their knowledge of the patient's pathology or disease process, familiarity with physical therapy interventions and alternatives, awareness of the standard of practice for treating that pathology, and the best available research evidence.[17] Proving that treatment is reasonable and necessary in documentation can be difficult. The therapist begins by integrating disablement concepts already discussed in Chapter 1 and integrating clinical problem solving. In addition to these principles, one must make sure the *reason* for implementing an intervention is provided in the documentation and the intervention is aimed at a specific problem(s) identified in the data. For example, the PT documents the following problems for a patient with lower back pain: (1) pain 8/10 when sitting, bending, and twisting, limiting work activities as mail handler; and (2) decreased spinal mobility including rotation, side bending, and forward flexion also limiting work activities. When documenting the interventions, the PT writes: "The patient will receive the following interventions: (1) modalities to control pain; and (2) spinal mobility exercises to restore range of motion, etc." This allows the reader to know *why* the intervention will be performed.

At regular intervals throughout the episode of care, the PT must use documentation to provide proof that interventions *continue* to be reasonable and necessary. To do this, the therapist not only summarizes clinically significant progress brought on by the interventions but also provides a list of remaining deficits or problems and a rationale for ongoing services, including new interventions that will be added. For the patient in the prior paragraph, on treatment day 6, the PT documents the following: "The patient's pain has decreased from 8/10 to 4/10 since initiating therapy. His spinal mobility has increased 20 degrees in all directions, thereby allowing improved work activities. We will progress to spinal stabilization exercises to further improve core strength and function at work."

When a patient is not improving as expected, justifying that care is reasonable and necessary is more challenging. The therapist must discern the reason why the patient is not improving. Perhaps he or she should change the intervention or maybe there are factors that are complicating the patient's progress. For example, the patient may have a secondary diagnosis that is hindering improvement or the patient may have a complicated social situation that is interfering with treatment. Another consideration is that the patient has reached his or her maximum potential for improvement and should be provided with a maintenance program. Whatever the reason for lack of improvement, or if there is a chronic condition, if the therapist chooses to continue, the documentation must be able to support that ongoing services are medically necessary and satisfy the reasonable and necessary conditions. In these more challenging cases, the therapist should integrate best available evidence, patient and/or family concerns, clinical judgment, and clinical problem solving in order to arrive at a decision and then he or she should articulate the clinical decision and supporting rationale in the documentation.

PROVIDE PROOF OF SKILLED CARE

One important aspect of the reasonable and necessary conditions is the need for "skilled services" or "skilled care." (See bullets 2 and 3 on pp 16 and 17). In addition to meeting other conditions for reasonable and necessary, the documentation provides proof that care provided to a patient is "skilled." Skilled services are those that have inherent complexity that, for safety and/or effectiveness, must be carried out *only* by or under the supervision of skilled nursing or skilled rehabilitation personnel to achieve patient safety and the medically desired outcome.[15] In other words, the patient requires a sophisticated and complex intervention that can be carried out safely and effectively only by a licensed PT or PTA.

This intervention may also require the unique judgment of a trained individual.

The patient's medical condition is a factor in deciding whether skilled services are needed. However, neither the diagnosis nor the prognosis should ever be the sole factor in determining whether a patient needs skilled services.[15] Rather, documentation must portray how or why the skills of the health care provider are needed. The therapist should describe the skills provided in the interventions as they occur or when he or she is planning to implement any new skilled interventions. Also, the therapist documents skills needed to maintain safety and effectiveness.

Consider the following 2 excerpts from a patient record and determine which one is more skilled.

1. The patient ambulated 50' with a wide-based quad cane and minimal assist × 1.

2. The patient ambulated 50' with a wide-based quad cane while the therapist provided physical assist and tactile cues to facilitate swing and prevent toe drag.

The second example shows how the unique skills of the therapist were utilized in the session and demonstrates the need for skilled gait training.

Services that are not skilled are considered palliative or maintenance. Maintenance services are those that are routine; promote the general health of the patient; "maintain" the patient's present status; and do not require the unique, complex, or sophisticated skills of a PT for safety and/or effectiveness.[15] An example is performance of an exercise program for a patient who wants to maintain motion or strength achieved in a formal physical therapy program. Maintenance therapy services can be performed by the patient through an independent home program or by an unlicensed individual, such as the family member or caregiver, who has received training from a skilled professional.

There are times, however, when maintenance services are allowed to be considered under skilled care. These include the following[15]:

- When the PT or PTA works with the patient and/or family to establish and provide instruction in a home exercise program prior to discharge from a facility

- When a PT evaluates a patient and establishes a home exercise maintenance program when no other services are provided (eg, a patient with osteoarthritis is referred to physical therapy for an examination and establishment of an aquatic therapy program. Following the examination, the PT works with the patient for 3 sessions to increase the patient's independence in performing the aquatic program).

- When the patient's safety may be jeopardized as in cases where the patient has a complex, unpredictable medical situation, multiple comorbidities complicating his or her situation, or when the result of the situation or intervention is unpredictable. This rule may apply to a patient who requires performing routine range of motion exercises, but presence of unstable or recent fractures allows the intervention to be considered under skilled care.

Of course, documentation must support or describe the need for the skilled intervention in these situations.

FACILITATE ADMINISTRATIVE DUTIES

In some clinics or health care systems, administrators use the physical therapy documentation to perform necessary administrative tasks. For example, in acute care hospitals, skilled nursing units, and inpatient rehabilitation settings, administrators use the documentation to identify the case mix groups in the facility. The case mix describes characteristics of the patients admitted to a particular unit or facility, which is required for establishing reimbursement parameters and for describing the type or severity of patients seen. The documentation informs the administrators regarding physical therapy utilization and during quality assurance activities. Other administrative uses include assessing the effectiveness and cost-effectiveness of services, strategic planning, and marketing.[18] Physical therapy documentation aids in our ability to analyze and study patient outcomes. Outcomes are defined as the end result of patient/client management.[1] Collection of outcome data is a growing area in physical therapy that is necessary for evidence-based practice. For example, analysis of patient outcomes can allow us to determine the effectiveness of physical therapy interventions.

SERVE AS A LEGAL RECORD OF CARE

Medical records are legal documents and any entries made into the medical record become part of that legal document. For this reason, it is important your documentation is accurate, legible, and depicts the patient's condition and the intervention appropriately and completely. Be aware that a patient's medical records can be subpoenaed and used as evidence in a variety of legal matters. These include motor vehicle accidents, worker's compensation or disability claims, and malpractice suits brought against you or other health care providers.

In malpractice lawsuits, documentation is the clinician's first line of defense.[19] Notes that are "clear, objective, thorough, and relevant make plaintiff's allegations of negligence more difficult to prove."[20(p2)] Good documentation can prevent a lawsuit, but poor documentation can be "powerful evidence in support of a suit, even when the accusations are frivolous."[5(p30)] Consider the following as a rule of thumb: If it is not documented, it did not happen. Following the guidelines for documentation in this text; recommendations set forth by the APTA, state and federal laws, and government agencies (eg, Medicare and Medicaid); and facility policies can help to protect you if you become involved in a malpractice lawsuit. Legal and

REVIEW QUESTIONS

1. List reasons for documenting in physical therapy.

   record patient/client management, communicate w/ others, demonstrate clinical problem solving, provide proof of skilled care

2. What aspects of patient/client management are included in documentation?

   referral, relevant pt. data, PT's assessment, all interventions provided, discharge summary

3. Explain how a PT's clinical problem solving can be reflected in his or her documentation.

   by documenting impairments, activity limitations, participation restrictions + describe adequacy of interventions used

4. What other individuals might be reviewing physical therapy documentation?

5. What information does a PTA gather from the PT's documentation?

6. How is documentation tied with reimbursement?

7. What are the criteria for determining if an intervention is reasonable and necessary?

8. What is meant by "medically necessary"?

9. How can a PT demonstrate medical necessity in a patient's record?

10. What is meant by the term *skilled care*?

11. How can a PT provide proof of skilled care in a patient's record?

12. Define maintenance.

13. List 2 examples of when maintenance therapy is considered skilled.

14. How does an administrator use documentation?

15. How is the documentation used in the legal system?

ethical issues regarding documentation are described more in the next chapter.

APPLICATION EXERCISES

Read through the following scenarios and discuss if the treatment would be considered maintenance or skilled. Give an explanation for your answer. If you choose maintenance, what are some things that you should do to initiate discontinuing treatment?

1. You are working with a patient in a nursing home who has severe Alzheimer's disease. Every afternoon, you take her for a walk through the hallways, around the building. She demonstrates weakness in her right ankle and there is a foot slap during the contact phase of gait. She can control it if given verbal cueing. You have been working with her for a month and you are not seeing any follow-through from one session to the next, and she has not progressed her distance or assistance needed in the last 2 weeks.

2. You have been doing some work for a home health agency in the evenings to make some extra money. The patient you are currently seeing has not shown improvement in the last week or so and the exercise program could be carried out by a family member. She is an 85-year-old woman with Parkinson disease who lives with her daughter. You are considering discharge when one day, the patient's daughter tells you that her mother enjoys having you come in and they really believe that you are helping.

3. You are working in a skilled nursing unit and you are assigned a patient who requires maximum assist for transfers due to a femur fracture and non–weight-bearing restrictions. The patient cannot participate in therapy due to lethargy and confusion.

4. You are working in an outpatient physical therapy clinic with a patient who has a frozen shoulder. She has been participating in therapy for about 6 weeks. During that time, she has made a substantial amount of progress. Over the last 2 weeks, her range of motion has started to plateau and she has resumed 90% of her functional activities. The patient attends therapy twice a week for passive stretching.

5. You are working on gait training with a patient who had a right CVA and has resultant left hemiplegia. While ambulating, you provide tactile and verbal cueing to the quadriceps to achieve full knee extension in late swing. The patient can respond to your cues about 50% of the time. This has improved over the last week and the patient requires less assistance than during the initial examination.

REFERENCES

1. American Physical Therapy Association. *Guide to Physical Therapist Practice*. 2nd ed. Alexandria, VA: APTA; 2003.
2. American Physical Therapy Association House of Delegates. Code of Ethics for the Physical Therapist HOD S06-09-07-12. http://www.apta.org/uploadedFiles/APTAorg/About_Us /Policies/Ethics/CodeofEthics.pdf. Accessed May 16, 2012.
3. Erickson ML, McKnight R. *Documentation Basics: A Guide for the PTA*. 2nd ed. Thorofare, NJ: SLACK Incorporated; 2012.
4. Arriaga R. Liability awareness. Stories from the front: documentation and clinical decision making: a real-life scenario illustrates some basic risk-management principles. *PT Magazine*. 2002;10(5):46-49.
5. Lewis DK. Do the write thing: document everything. *PT Magazine*. 2002;10(7):30-34.
6. Redgate N, Foto M. Pay by the rules: avoid Medicare audits and reduce payment denials with a sound strategy and proper documentation. *Phys Ther Prod*. 2003;October/November:28–30.
7. Baeten AM. Documentation: the reviewer perspective. *Top Geriatr Rehabil*. 1997;13(1):14-22.
8. Inaba M, Jones SL. Medical documentation for third-party payers. *Phys Ther*. 1977;57:791-794.
9. American Physical Therapy Association. Guidelines: Physical Therapy Documentation of Patient/Client Management. http://www.apta.org/uploadedFiles/APTAorg/About_Us /Policies/BOD/Practice/DocumentationPatientClientMgmt .pdf. Accessed May 16, 2012.
10. American Physical Therapy Association. Defensible documentation. http://www.apta.org/Documentation/Defensible Documentation/. Accessed May 16, 2012.
11. Centers for Medicare & Medicaid Services. Covered medical and other health services. *Medicare Benefit Policy Manual*. Publication 100-02. http://www.cms.gov/Regulations-and -Guidance/Guidance/Manuals/Downloads/bp102c15.pdf. Accessed May 16, 2012.
12. Centers for Medicare & Medicaid Services. Home health services. *Medicare Benefit Policy Manual*. Publication 100-02. http://www.cms.gov/Regulations-and-Guidance/Guidance /Manuals/Downloads/bp102c07.pdf. Accessed May 16, 2012.
13. Centers for Medicare & Medicaid Services. Inpatient hospital services covered under part A. *Medicare Benefit Policy Manual*. Publication 100-02. http://www.cms .gov/Regulations-and-Guidance/Guidance/Manuals /Downloads/bp102c01.pdf. Accessed May 16, 2012.
14. Centers for Medicare & Medicaid Services. Comprehensive outpatient rehabilitation facility (CORF) coverage. *Medicare Benefit Policy Manual*. Publication 100-02. http://www .cms.gov/Regulations-and-Guidance/Guidance/Manuals /Downloads/bp102c12.pdf. Accessed May 16, 2012.
15. Centers for Medicare & Medicaid Services. Coverage of extended care (SNF) services under hospital insurance. *Medicare Benefit Policy Manual*. Publication 100-02. http: //www.cms.gov/Regulations-and-Guidance/Guidance /Manuals/Downloads/bp102c08.pdf. Accessed May 16, 2012.
16. Centers for Medicare & Medicaid Services. Medicare glossary definition for medically necessary. http://www .medicare.gov/Glossary/m.html. Accessed May 16, 2012.
17. Moorhead JF, Clifford J. Determining medical necessity of outpatient physical therapy services. *Am J Med Qual*. 1992;7(3):81-84.
18. Shamus E, Stern D. *Effective Documentation for Physical Therapy Professionals*. 2nd ed. New York, NY: McGraw-Hill Companies Inc; 2011.
19. Schunk CR. Liability awareness. Advice for the new physical therapist: here are some keys to avoiding risk once you've made the transition from student to practitioner. *PT Magazine*. 2001;9(11):24-26.
20. Lewis DK. Lessons from COURT. *HPSO Risk Advisor*. 2000;3(2). www.hpso.com. Accessed June 6, 2006.

Chapter 3

Ethical and Regulatory Issues in Physical Therapy Documentation

Ralph R. Utzman, PT, MPH, PhD

CHAPTER OUTLINE

Law, Regulation, and Policy
Informed Consent
Malpractice and Risk Management
Patient Safety and Quality of Care
Confidentiality
Reimbursement, Fraud, and Abuse

CHAPTER OBJECTIVES

Upon completion of this chapter, the reader will be able to:

1. Compare and contrast law, regulation, and policy.
2. Describe how the APTA's *Code of Ethics for the Physical Therapist* addresses documentation-related issues, such as informed consent, confidentiality, reimbursement, fraud, and abuse.
3. Define informed consent.
4. Discuss how documentation serves as a risk-management tool.
5. Describe the function of the medical record as a communication tool to improve patient safety and quality of care.
6. Describe the purpose of incident reports and identify how incident reports should be filed.
7. Describe how the *Health Insurance Portability and Accountability Act* safeguards patient privacy.

Erickson ML, Utzman RR, McKnight R. *Physical Therapy Documentation:*
From Examination to Outcome, Second Edition (pp 21-27).
© 2014 SLACK Incorporated.

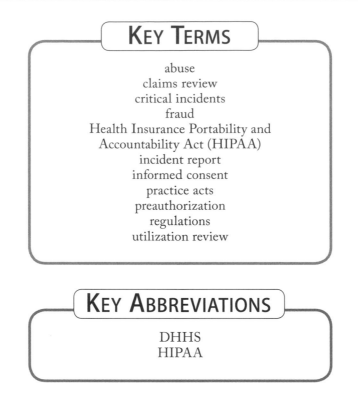

KEY TERMS

abuse
claims review
critical incidents
fraud
Health Insurance Portability and
Accountability Act (HIPAA)
incident report
informed consent
practice acts
preauthorization
regulations
utilization review

KEY ABBREVIATIONS

DHHS
HIPAA

The previous chapter described the clinical problem-solving skills PTs use to provide patient care. To solve patient problems, PTs access, record, and transmit a wide variety of patients' medical, personal, and social information. The primary vehicle for this information is the medical record, which is itself a legal document. Therefore, PT practice requires careful attention to ethical principles and compliance with laws and regulations related to documentation and the medical record.

This chapter introduces readers to ethical, legal, and regulatory issues related to clinical documentation. This chapter is not intended as a substitute for professional legal advice. Many health care facilities employ or retain licensed attorneys to assist with managing legal risks associated with providing health care. Other facilities, as well as therapists in private practice, can obtain legal advice from the insurance company from whom they purchase malpractice/liability coverage. Many organizations have compliance officers or departments that assist health care providers in understanding and following current regulations. Readers are urged to seek advice from one of these sources when confronted with specific questions in clinical practice.

LAW, REGULATION, AND POLICY

Laws are governmental statements of what we must do. They are developed by votes of Congress, state legislatures, or county/municipal governments. Laws can also result from court cases in which a decision by a judge or jury sets a precedent for future cases. Laws often delegate oversight of a law to a government agency or regulatory body. This government agency may then write regulations, or rules,

that state how the intent of the law is to be carried out. Such regulations typically carry the force of law.

For example, consider state laws that govern PT practice. In all 50 states, laws exist that define what physical therapy is and who can practice physical therapy. These laws, which are enacted by state legislatures, are commonly known as physical therapy practice acts. In most states, these practice acts include provisions for a licensure board, which is a government agency that oversees the practice of physical therapy. The licensure board, in turn, may write regulations that further describe parameters of practice. If a therapist fails to comply with either the practice act or regulations, the licensing board may suspend or revoke the therapist's license to practice.

Although laws and regulations are written by the government and its agencies, policies are rules written by nongovernmental organizations. Such organizations include professional associations (eg, APTA) or accrediting bodies (eg, The Joint Commission). Health care organizations, such as hospitals and clinics, also develop policies that govern their employees. A primary purpose of organizational policy is to standardize the actions and behaviors of members of that organization. Organizational policies can also serve to communicate the values and philosophies that guide members' behaviors.

The APTA has several policies related to documentation of physical therapy care. The APTA's *Guidelines for Physical Therapy Documentation of Patient/Client Management*[1] is reprinted in Appendix A. This document outlines the profession's standards for documentation. The *Guidelines* are rooted in a broader APTA document, the *Code of Ethics for the Physical Therapist*.[2]

The *Code of Ethics for the Physical Therapist* consists of 8 principles that are broad statements of PTs' responsibilities.[2] Each of the 8 principles includes 2 or more additional statements that further define the therapist's responsibilities in that particular area. Out of the 8 main principles, 5 specifically address issues related to documentation and communication with other health care personnel. The following sections of this chapter address specific ethical and legal issues related to documentation, with references to the *Code of Ethics* and key regulations as applicable.

INFORMED CONSENT

Informed consent refers to the right of the patient to make his or her own decisions about the care he or she receives. Principle 2C of the *Code of Ethics* states, "PT shall provide the information necessary to allow patients . . . to make informed decisions about physical therapy care. . . . "[2] In order to make a decision, the patient needs to know what treatment is being recommended; the potential benefits, costs, and risks of that treatment; and what alternatives exist. The best way for a PT to accomplish this is to talk with the patient, then document the outcome of the discussion. See Chapter 8 for examples.

Even though physical therapy care is typically conservative and presents low risks to patients compared with surgery and medications, no treatment is completely free of risk. Suppose that a therapist performs a stretching technique on a patient following tendon repair surgery. Even though an appropriate amount of time has elapsed since the surgery, and the patient's surgeon has verified that gentle stretching may begin, there is still a small chance that even gentle stretching may cause the repaired tendon to rupture. The therapist should explain this, along with other treatment alternatives, to the patient before beginning the treatment session. If the therapist provides the treatment and the repaired tendon ruptures, the therapist may face a malpractice lawsuit. The therapist's best defense is careful documentation of the patient's clinical status, the patient's informed consent to the stretching procedure, and the treatment and follow-up provided.

MALPRACTICE AND RISK MANAGEMENT

Any time a PT provides care to a patient, the therapist is taking a legal risk. Malpractice lawsuits can result from a variety of issues, including the following:

- Improper performance of therapeutic exercise or manual therapy
- Injury from modalities, such as hot packs or electrical stimulation
- Failure to adequately supervise/monitor patients and support personnel
- Improper management or treatment of the patient (eg, performing inappropriate treatment techniques)

- Failure to perform appropriate tests/measures
- Injuries caused by equipment or falls caused by cluttered environment[3]

Many facilities employ risk managers, or use risk management committees or departments, whose responsibilities include minimizing potential risks for health care providers involved with patient/client management. In a private practice, the owner may serve as the risk manager. Besides providing training for clinicians on managing legal risks, these individuals or groups investigate complaints or concerns as they are brought forth, either by patients or providers. An important aspect of their investigation is examining the medical record and other available documentation. Good documentation is the cornerstone of good risk management, allowing risk managers to determine if quality care standards were met and future risks are avoided.

According to a report prepared by the Agency for Healthcare Research and Quality, critical incidents include adverse events that result in patient harm or have potential to cause harm but do not.[4] For instance, a therapist may discover that an electrical stimulation machine is malfunctioning. Depending on the nature of the malfunction and when it was discovered, the patient may or may not suffer a burn. When an adverse event leads to patient injury, the therapist should record the objective facts regarding the incident in the medical record. These facts should include information regarding the injury, instructions given to the patient, communication of the incident with referring physicians or other health care providers, and any follow-up care provided to the patient.

Besides documenting critical incidents in the medical record, the therapist should also file an incident report. Incident reports are used to document "errors and departures from expected procedures or outcomes."[4(p47)] Incident reports serve as a tool for improving care by identifying and investigating problems as they arise.[4] Incident reports also provide an internal account in case legal action results from the adverse event.[5] Incident reports should be filed with your facility's risk management department or malpractice/liability insurer. Incident reports are used for administrative and training purposes. In many states, incident reports are protected from release to the plaintiff's attorneys because they are considered internal quality improvement documents, privileged communication between the clinician and his or her attorney, or both.[5] Therefore, they should not be filed with or mentioned in the medical record.[5,6]

[handwritten: Mention incident not incident report in documentation]

PATIENT SAFETY AND QUALITY OF CARE

Principle 3 of the *Code of Ethics* states, "PTs shall be accountable for making sound professional judgments."[2] Subitems included with this principle state that the PT is independently responsible (rather than a referring physician or facility administrator) for the decisions he or she makes, that he or she is responsible for using the best scientific evidence to inform those decisions, and that clinical judgments must be communicated clearly with peers, subordinates (ie, PTAs), and other health care providers.[2] The primary method for communicating professional judgment and decisions is the medical record. The reader of physical therapy documentation should be able to identify the key findings of the physical therapy examination, the rationale for the plan of care, any precautions to be followed, and the patient's response to treatment.

The medical record was originally designed as a mechanism to remind the individual health care provider of the treatment provided to date. For PTs, accurately recalling the precautions, objective measurements, and exercise programs of multiple patients over time would be nearly impossible. Communicating this information to coworkers is critical. Consider the patients of a PT who is called away from the clinic unexpectedly; another therapist agrees to provide care for these patients in his or her absence. Without well-written medical records, the therapist filling in for the absent colleague would have no way to know what treatments had been provided previously, how the patients had responded, and what future treatments were planned. In this situation, the covering therapist would not be able to provide safe, effective treatment to the patients.

As the health care system has become increasingly specialized and complex, communication between physicians, therapists, nurses, and others has become increasingly important. Patients with complex medical conditions, limitations, and precautions are frequently referred to physical therapy. PTs are often supported by PTAs, who provide elements of the plan of care with supervision from the PT. In some settings and jurisdictions, the supervising PT need not always be on-site while the assistant is providing treatment. In the absence of good documentation, communication of key information is likely to be missed, leading to poor quality of care and potential harm to the patient.

For example, consider the case of an older woman who has been admitted to a skilled nursing facility following surgical repair of a proximal femur fracture. The surgeon has referred the patient for physical therapy with a precaution that the patient should bear no more than 10% of her body weight on the involved lower extremity. Although the referral has been transmitted to the PT, she neglects to document the precaution in her initial note and plan of care. Subsequent treatment sessions are provided by a PTA. After several treatment sessions, the patient complains of increased hip and thigh pain in the involved extremity. The patient's family, concerned about the patient's increased pain, contacts the surgeon, who orders a radiograph. The radiograph reveals that the surgical repair of the fracture has failed and the patient requires further surgery. Because the PT did not document the weight-bearing restriction, the medical record does not reflect professional judgment by the PT. The therapist is responsible for the care provided by the assistant (*Code of Ethics* item 5B[2]), and with no clear documentation of the instructions provided to the assistant, the therapist may be found liable for the patient's poor clinical outcome.

Better patient outcomes can be achieved through improved documentation practices. Consider another patient with a similar diagnosis and referral. When admitted to the skilled nursing facility, the therapist carefully documents the post-surgical precautions. The patient is somewhat confused and has difficulty following instructions during the initial examination. The therapist documents this and carefully outlines a plan of care and instructions for the assistant. During subsequent treatments, the assistant notes the patient's difficulty in maintaining the weight-bearing restrictions and appropriately limits progression of the patient's ambulation during treatment sessions. When reviewing the medical record prior to the next supervisory visit, the PT notes the assistant's concerns as well as reports from nursing staff that the patient has been getting out of bed at night without assistance. The therapist notifies the surgeon and collaborates with the assistant and nursing staff regarding strategies to progress the patient's mobility safely. Together with the patient's family, the staff develops a plan to reduce the risk of the patient getting out of bed at night by herself. These plans and the patient's progress are carefully documented and the patient gradually learns to use her walker safely without reinjuring herself. Although the patient stays in the facility for several days longer than initially expected, she returns home with her family without the need for further surgery.

CONFIDENTIALITY

Principle 2E of the *Code of Ethics* states that PTs must "protect confidential patient/client information and may disclose confidential information . . . only when allowed or as required by law."[2] This principle underscores the fact that PTs have access to a host of sensitive information about patients. Medical records may contain information about genetics, mental health, substance abuse, infectious diseases, and more. Some patients prefer to not share basic information, such as age or weight, even with close relatives. Medical records may include identifying data that can be exploited by identity thieves. Because medical records contain such sensitive data, they should be viewed as an extension of the individual and treated with the same respect and care expected by the patient.

Because of a series of high-profile breaches of patient confidentiality, the issue was included in the landmark federal law known as the Health Insurance Portability and Accountability Act (HIPAA) of 1996. Title I of HIPAA allows workers to maintain their insurance coverage when they change jobs. Title II focuses on preventing fraud and abuse and required the US Department of Health and Human Services (DHHS) to establish rules for safeguarding the privacy of patients' personal health information.

The final privacy rule developed by DHHS went into effect on April 14, 2003. Health care providers, health insurance plans, and health information clearinghouses are subject to the rule if they hold or transmit protected health information in any form—oral, written, facsimile, or electronic. Protected health information includes all personal health information, including medical records and other identifiable health information.[6] Electronic media refers to the Internet, intranets and extranets, leased lines,

<table>
<tr><td colspan="1">

Table 3-1
Data to Be Removed to "Deidentify" Patient Records

1. Names
2. All elements of address smaller than the state
3. All elements of dates related to the patient (eg, birth date, death date, admission/discharge date) except the year
4. Phone numbers
5. Facsimile numbers
6. Electronic mail addresses
7. Social security numbers
8. Medical record numbers
9. Insurance numbers
10. Account numbers
11. Certificate/license numbers
12. Vehicle identification, registration, and license plate numbers
13. Identifiers (serial numbers) of medical devices
14. Internet addresses (URLs)
15. Internet protocol (IP) address numbers
16. Fingerprints, voice prints, and other biometric data
17. Full-face photographs or similar images that could be used to identify the patient
18. Any other unique identifier, code, or characteristic

</td></tr>
</table>

Reprinted from National Institutes of Health, US Department of Health and Human Services. How can covered entities use and disclose protected health information for research and comply with the privacy rule? http://privacyruleandresearch.nih.gov/pr_08.asp#8a. Accessed November 1, 2012.

dial-up lines, private networks, or transmissions occurring through magnetic tape, disk, or compact disk.[7] Under the privacy rule, patients are granted several rights, including the following:

- The right to read and get copies of their own medical records
- The right to make amendments to their own medical records
- The right to know who has access to their medical records
- The right to give written permission prior to disclosure of their personal health information
- The right to file a complaint when they believe their privacy is not being protected[8]

The privacy rule allows health care providers to share information without written consent in circumstances that relate to routine care of the patient. Such circumstances would include providing information to a physician or other health care provider involved in the patient's care or providing copies of medical records to insurance companies for reimbursement purposes.[9] Such disclosures should provide only the minimum information necessary to accomplish the purpose.[10]

Under the HIPAA privacy rule, health care providers must obtain consent prior to releasing patients' protected health information for other reasons, such as marketing or research.[8] For instance, if a PT or student is writing a case report on a patient, the author must obtain patient consent first. However, the material may be used without consent if it is first "de-identified." This means that any information that could potentially be used to identify the patient must be removed. The rule lists 18 elements that must be removed. In addition, the author would need to be sure that the patient could not be identified in any way from the remaining information.[11] The 18 elements that must be removed are listed in Table 3-1.[11] These elements may be removed electronically or manually. Research protocols must be designed in ways that safeguard patient privacy and these methods must be approved by an institutional review board.[11]

The privacy rule requires health care facilities to provide training related to patient privacy safeguards to their employees. Facilities are also required to designate a privacy officer to oversee employee training and overall implementation of privacy safeguards.[6] Many states have laws regarding privacy of personal health information. If the state law is more stringent than the HIPAA privacy rule, the state law supersedes HIPAA.[8]

REIMBURSEMENT, FRAUD, AND ABUSE

As noted in previous chapters, medical records are routinely used for insurance reimbursement purposes. Medical records may be reviewed for preauthorization, or approval for payment prior to delivery of nonemergency health care services. Medical records may be subject to utilization review during the course of care to make sure appropriate care is being provided. Claims review may be used after services are provided to compare the medical record to the final bill to make a final determination regarding whether or not services provided are to be reimbursed.

Principle 7B of the *Code of Ethics* states that "PTs shall seek remuneration as is deserved and reasonable . . .."[2] Further, Item 4A states that "PTs shall provide truthful, accurate, and relevant information and shall not make misleading representations."[2] Finally, item 5A states that PTs must comply with laws and regulations.[2] Taken together, the items from the *Code* prohibit the PT from engaging in reimbursement fraud and abuse. Insurance fraud can be defined as billing a third-party payer for services that were never provided or billing for an item or service that is reimbursed at a higher rate than the service that was actually provided.[12] Fraud is a crime and is punishable by law. Another improper billing procedure is abuse. Abuse occurs when a provider bills for items that are not covered or misuses billing codes.[12] Abuse differs from fraud in that fraud is intentional, whereas abuse often results from unintended billing errors or poor awareness of proper billing and coding procedures. In 2009, DHHS and the Department of Justice created a joint task force to combat Medicare and Medicaid fraud and abuse.[13] Individual states will also investigate claims of fraud and abuse of private insurance plans.

In order to avoid accusations of abuse, PTs should stay abreast of current reimbursement and coding guidelines. Accurate billing with corresponding documentation can help prevent fraud accusations. According to *Code of Ethics* Principle 7E, PTs have a duty to understand billing and coding for physical therapy services.[2] More detail on reimbursement is provided in Chapter 12.

REVIEW QUESTIONS

1. What are the differences between laws, regulations, and policies? What are the similarities?

2. What functions do state boards of physical therapy serve?

3. Describe how the medical record serves as a tool for risk management.
   It allows risk managers to assess the quality of care and future implications of interventions

4. What is informed consent? How should consent be documented in the medical record?
   "right of the pt. to make his/her own decisions about his/her care" PT should document the outcome of the risk discussion

5. What are the purposes of the HIPAA privacy rule?
   Pts. have the right to their own medical records & the right to decide if/how their PHI is shared

6. What types of occurrences should be documented on incident reports? How and where should incident reports be filed? *errors & departures from expected procedures - Should be filed w/ facility's risk management dept. or malpractice/ liability insurer after a critical incident*

APPLICATION EXERCISES

1. Obtain copies of the physical therapy practice act (statutory law) and practice rules/regulations for your state. Review the documents and answer the following questions.

   a. What is the scope of practice of a PT? A PTA? Are there any limitations regarding what a PTA is allowed to document compared to a PT?

   b. What are the rules for supervising PTAs and other support personnel?

   c. Is a referral required for a patient to receive physical therapy services? If so, who may refer? If there are provisions for direct access (evaluation/treatment without referral), are there any limitations or restrictions?

   d. What rules apply to authenticating (signing) entries in the medical record? What initials should follow the PTs name? If the therapist holds a Doctor of Physical Therapy degree, may he or she use this designator in the medical record? Is the therapist required to include his or her license number?

    e. What are the potential consequences for practice inconsistent with the practice act or rules/regulations?

2. Review your organization's policies and procedures for documentation. Do these policies coincide with APTA's *Guidelines for Physical Therapy Documentation of Patient/Client Management* (Appendix A)?

3. Review your organization's policies for patient confidentiality.

    a. How is the patient notified of his or her rights?

    b. How may a patient request copies of his or her medical record?

    c. How does the organization restrict access to the medical record?

    d. If a patient's confidentiality is breached, how would the facility respond? What sanctions would be taken against an employee who breaches patient confidentiality?

REFERENCES

1. American Physical Therapy Association. Guidelines: Physical therapy documentation of patient/client management. http://www.apta.org/uploadedFiles/APTAorg/About_Us/Policies/BOD/Practice/DocumentationPatientClientMgmt.pdf. Accessed November 1, 2012.

2. American Physical Therapy Association. Code of ethics for the physical therapist. http://www.apta.org/uploadedFiles/APTAorg/About_Us/Policies/HOD/Ethics/CodeofEthics.pdf. Accessed November 1, 2012.

3. Health Providers Service Organization. Physical therapy liability 2001–2010. http://www.hpso.com/pdfs/db/CNA_CLS_PTreport_final_011312.pdf?fileName=CNA_CLS_PTreport_final_011312.pdf&folder=pdfs/db&isLiveStr=Y. Accessed November 1, 2012.

4. Wald H, Shojania KG. Incident reporting. In: Shojania KG, Duncan BW, McDonald KM, Wachter RM, eds. *Making Health Care Safer: A Critical Analysis of Patient Safety Practices.* Rockville, MD: Agency for Healthcare Research and Quality; 2001. AHRQ publication 01-E058. https://www.premierinc.com/safety/topics/patient_safety/downloads/23_AHRQ_evidence_report_43.pdf. Accessed April 27, 2013.

5. Scott RW. Clinical patient care documentation methods and management. In: *Legal, Ethical, and Practical Aspects of Patient Care Documentation.* 4th ed. Burlington, MA: Jones & Bartlett Learning; 2013:35–92.

6. Nosse LJ, Friberg DG, Kovacek PR. Managing risk. In: *Managerial and Supervisory Principles for Physical Therapists.* 2nd ed. Baltimore, MD: Lippincott Williams & Wilkins; 2005:458–479.

7. Ravitz KS. The HIPAA privacy final modified rule. *PT-Magazine of Physical Therapy.* 2002;10(11):21-25.

8. Office of Civil Rights, US Department of Health and Human Services. Summary of the HIPAA privacy rule. http://www.hhs.gov/ocr/privacy/hipaa/understanding/summary/index.html. Accessed November 1, 2012.

9. Office of Civil Rights, US Department of Health and Human Services. Incidental uses and disclosures. http://www.hhs.gov/ocr/privacy/hipaa/understanding/coveredentities/incidentalusesanddisclosures.html. Accessed November 1, 2012.

10. Office of Civil Rights, US Department of Health and Human Services. Minimum necessary requirement. http://www.hhs.gov/ocr/privacy/hipaa/understanding/coveredentities/minimumnecessary.html. Accessed November 1, 2012.

11. National Institutes of Health, US Department of Health and Human Services. How can covered entities use and disclose protected health information for research and comply with the privacy rule? http://privacyrule andresearch.nih.gov/pr_08.asp#8a. Accessed November 1, 2012.

12. Centers for Medicare & Medicaid Services. CMS glossary. http://www.cms.gov/apps/glossary/default.asp?Letter=F&Language=English. Accessed November 1, 2012.

13. US Department of Health and Human Services and US Department of Justice. HEAT task force. http://www.stopmedicarefraud.gov/aboutfraud/heattaskforce/index.html. Accessed November 1, 2012.

Chapter 4

Documenting Patient/Client Management
An Overview

Mia L. Erickson, PT, EdD, CHT, ATC and Rebecca McKnight, PT, MS

CHAPTER OUTLINE

CHAPTER OBJECTIVES

Upon completion of this chapter, the reader will be able to:
1. Describe components of the Patient/Client Management Model.
2. List requirements for documenting the initial visit with a patient.
3. Differentiate between the examination and evaluation according to the Patient/Client Management Model.
4. Realize the differing definitions for "evaluation."
5. Realize the importance of documenting function and impairments.
6. List information that should be included in the assessment and plan portions of the initial documentation.

Erickson ML, Utzman RR, McKnight R. *Physical Therapy Documentation:*
From Examination to Outcome, Second Edition (pp 29-40).
© 2014 SLACK Incorporated.

7. Compare and contrast interim (or treatment) notes and progress reports.
8. Differentiate between a short-term and a long-term goal.
9. Describe information to be included in a discharge note, or summary.
10. Differentiate between discharge and discontinuation.

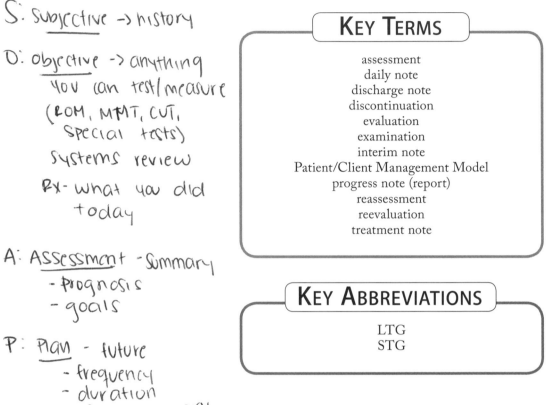

S: Subjective -> history

D: objective -> anything
   you can test/measure
   (ROM, MMT, CUT,
   special tests)
   systems review

Rx- what you did
    today

A: Assessment - Summary
   - prognosis
   - goals

P: Plan - future
   - frequency
   - duration
   - Rx - treatment

KEY TERMS

assessment
daily note
discharge note
discontinuation
evaluation
examination
interim note
Patient/Client Management Model
progress note (report)
reassessment
reevaluation
treatment note

KEY ABBREVIATIONS

LTG
STG

PATIENT/CLIENT MANAGEMENT

The *Guide to Physical Therapist Practice*[1] defines the role of the PT with regard to patient care through the Patient/Client Management Model. The Patient/Client Management Model consists of 5 elements, or components, that include examination, evaluation, diagnosis, prognosis, and intervention. The 5 components ultimately lead to an outcome, or end result. During the initial patient encounter, the PT performs and documents the initial examination and evaluation. The Patient/Client Management Model differentiates examination from evaluation in that the *examination* is the process of screening and performing tests and measures.[1] During this phase, the PT obtains the patient history, performs a systems review or screening of various body systems, and performs specific tests and measures.[1] The Patient/Client Management Model then defines the *evaluation* as a process by which the PT synthesizes data from the examination and arrives at a diagnosis, prognosis, and plan for intervention.[1] Although the Patient/Client Management Model clearly differentiates between the terms and processes of examination and evaluation, the terms are often used synonymously. Additionally, in the clinical setting, they are often collectively known as "the

initial evaluation." Furthermore, Centers for Medicare & Medicaid Services (CMS) defines evaluation as[2(p150)]:

a separately payable comprehensive service provided by a (physical therapist), that requires professional skills to make clinical judgments about conditions for which services are indicated based on objective measurements and subjective evaluations of patient performance and functional abilities. Evaluation is warranted eg, for a new diagnosis or when a condition is treated in a new setting. These evaluative judgments are essential to development of the plan of care, including goals and the selection of interventions.

Because there are many definitions for the terms *examination* and *evaluation*, there is basis for confusion. In order to be consistent with the *Guide to Physical Therapist Practice* and the Patient/Client Management Model, throughout this text, we refer to *examination* as the process of collecting patient-related data and the *evaluation* as the process of clinical decision making that occurs following the examination. The evaluation then in turn allows the PT to determine the patient's diagnosis. This could be a medical diagnosis and/or a physical therapy or movement diagnosis. A physical therapy or movement diagnosis is a label used to describe the patient's movement-related dysfunction or disorder(s) and it often provides the target for which future interventions are aimed.

The PT also arrives at a prognosis. This is where he or she predicts or makes a clinical judgment regarding the patient's final outcome. The intervention is then determined and includes a comprehensive plan for what the therapist plans to do to affect the physical therapy or movement dysfunction(s).

DOCUMENTING THE INITIAL PATIENT ENCOUNTER
longest note

Subjective and Objective Data

At the onset of the initial patient encounter, the PT performs the examination by collecting and recording subjective and objective data regarding the patient's current and prior medical and functional status. These initial subjective and objective data include the patient history, systems review, and specific tests and measures. Subjective data, or the patient history, come from the patient, a family member, or a caregiver. Subjective data include the history of the present illness (HPI), mechanism of injury (MOI), date of injury (DOI) or onset date, prior medical history (PMH), chief complaints (C/C), current *and* prior level of function, information regarding the patient's lifestyle (L/S) such as living environment or situation, and the patient's goals for physical therapy, to name a few (see Example 4-1). Both the *Guide to Physical Therapist Practice* and the *Guidelines for Physical Therapy Documentation of Patient/Client Management*[3] (see Appendix A) provide examples of typical data gathered during the history-taking portion of the examination. More information on recording subjective data is provided in Chapter 7.

After obtaining the patient history, the PT collects objective data through (1) a review of systems and (2) physical therapy tests and measures. During a review of systems, or systems review, the PT assesses the patient's overall condition by grossly screening the cardiovascular and pulmonary (ie, heart rate, blood pressure, respiratory rate), integumentary, musculoskeletal, and neuromuscular systems. The PT also screens the patient's cognitive and communication abilities, affect, language, and learning style(s) during the systems review.[3] The PT then records the type of screening(s) completed and the results.

Based on information gleaned during the review of systems, the PT selects and performs more specific tests and measures to further examine the patient's status. These more specific tests and measures allow the PT to accurately pinpoint and measure physical therapy impairments, activity limitations, and participation restrictions in life roles and tasks. Performing and recording these measurements are crucial for establishing the physical therapy diagnosis, prognosis, and intervention plan.

The PT assesses and documents patient impairments such as joint range of motion, muscle strength, sensation, circulation, limb circumference, and balance. But the examination must go beyond the impairment level so the PT can see how the impairments are influencing the patient's day-to-day life. The therapist assesses patient function using performance-based measures that require the patient to perform functional tasks or using self-report measures that require the patient to complete a questionnaire, rating his or her overall performance on a set of functional tasks. Examining and documenting functional status provides more specific, contextual information regarding the impact of the pathologies and impairments on the patient's life roles and normal activities. We know from Chapter 1 that the mere presence of impairment does not always translate to functional loss. Furthermore, individuals reviewing medical records often deem the patient's functional status as being more meaningful than documentation of impairments alone. These initial impairment and functional data provide baseline measurements to which future data are compared to determine patient progress (see Example 4-1).[4] The *Guide to Physical Therapist Practice* and the *Guidelines for Physical Therapy Documentation of Patient/Client Management* (see Appendix A) provide a list of measures included in the systems review and tests and measures portion of the examination. More information on recording objective data is provided in Chapter 8.

The PT uses data collected in the history, review of systems, and tests and measures to make the clinical decisions needed to arrive at an intervention plan. Again, according to the Patient/Client Management Model, this clinical judgment is known as the *evaluation*.[1] You may also hear this process referred to as the impression or assessment. Recall that, according to the Patient/Client Management Model, the evaluation is actually a thought process, or clinical problem-solving process, whereby the PT considers all data gathered to establish the physical therapy diagnosis, the patient's prognosis, and the intervention plan.[1,5] In using the SOAP (subjective, objective, assessment, and plan) documentation format, the PT documents these latter aspects of the initial encounter in the assessment and plan (see Figure 4-1).

The Assessment and Plan

A Brief Summary of the Patient That Includes the Diagnosis

In the summary, the PT provides an overview of the patient and often includes the medical diagnosis, synthesizes the exam findings, and describes how the impairments may be contributing to or causing functional or activity limitations and participation restrictions. This section answers the question: "What is wrong with this patient?" The medical diagnosis can take many forms. Many PTs choose to use the medical diagnosis and/or the ICD-9 code and integrate it into the summary statement(s). This section also includes the physical therapy or movement diagnosis that can be taken from a practice pattern from the *Guide to Physical Therapist Practice* (see Appendix B). Alternatively, the PT may choose to describe the patient's movement dysfunction in his or her own words by describing how the impairments are contributing to the patient's functional problems. Any of these are appropriate. Finally, this aspect of documentation also includes a problem list that calls attention to the patient's specific impairments, activity limitations, and participation restrictions identified in the examination that will be addressed during the physical therapy episode of care (Figure 4-1).

Example 4-1. Example of Initial Patient Documentation

Patient name: Becky Smith
Date of service: August 1, 2012
Date of injury: July 4, 2012; 10:00 a.m.
Referral: Referred to PT for "shoulder and elbow PROM, sling on at all other times" by Dr. John Smith

Subjective: Patient history: 62 y.o. white, right-hand dominant woman, 4 weeks s/p fall from chair while changing light bulb when she sustained a (R) spiral humerus fracture. Immediately underwent ORIF and was placed in a sling. Saw the physician yesterday and was referred to PT. She returns to the physician in 2 weeks. She is hoping to have the sling discontinued at that time. PMH is unremarkable. Patient is a nonsmoker and reports being in good health. She had a hysterectomy 15 years ago.

C/C: Pain 6/10 with motion of the (R) arm movements and difficulty performing self-care skills because of decreased ability to use her (R) arm. Reports using over-the-counter ibuprofen for pain.

L/S: Patient lives in 2-story home with her husband. She has 2 grown children living nearby who can provide assistance. She is a retired teacher who substitute-teaches occasionally. Before the injury she states that she was very active including playing recreational tennis and walking daily. She has been unable to perform normal ADL including self-care, home management, driving, or exercising since the injury.

Patient's Goal: Return to her normal active lifestyle.

Objective: Systems Review: Cardiopulmonary system: HR: 88, BP 128/88, RR 10. Integumentary system: Incision present but healed. Musculoskeletal system: Patient is 5' 7" and 155#. She ambulated into the clinic without difficulty. Impaired (R) UE ROM. Neuromuscular system: Gross sensation to light touch in (B) UEs is intact. Communication/Cognition: Not impaired.

Tests and measures: Capillary refill: Intact Integumentary integrity: Immature adhered scar present along posterior humerus, dry, hypersensitive to touch, raised ~1-2 mm. Strength: (L) UE 5/5; (R) UE N/A this visit because of surgery. PROM: (R) shoulder: flexion 95° abduction 90° ER 35° IR 50°; elbow: –10/100°. AROM: cervical WNL; (R) wrist and hand WNL; (L) shoulder: flexion 160° abduction 160° ER 90° IR 70°; elbow 0/140°.

Functional assessment: DASH questionnaire score 84/100, see attached; requires assistance with ADL including hygiene, dressing, and bathing; unable to complete home management tasks, drive, work, or participate in normal recreational activities (ie, tennis, walking program).

Assessment and plan: 62 y.o. right-hand dominant woman 4 weeks s/p ORIF (R) humerus (ICD-9 code: 812) referred for shoulder and elbow PROM to dominant extremity; she presents with s/s of Musculoskeletal Practice Pattern G; ROM limitations in place by surgeon to protect healing fracture in the dominant extremity have significantly limited her ability to perform (I) self-care, hygiene, reaching, home tasks, work activities, recreational activities, or driving.

Problem list: Impairments: 1) decreased ROM (R) UE; 2) decreased strength (R) UE; 3) adhered scar; 4) pain 6/10. Function: 1) DASH score 84/100 indicating 84% disability; 2) requires assistance with ADL; 3) unable to perform normal life roles including reaching, home management tasks, driving, work activities, and recreational activities.

Prognosis: Patient has good social support and is motivated, demonstrating good potential to return to normal lifestyle and to meet established goals. No complicating factors identified at this time.

Discharge Goals (In 8 weeks, the patient will demonstrate):

1. AROM (R) UE 90%-100% of (L) to allow patient to perform ADL, reaching, driving, work, and recreational activities
2. Strength (R) 4 to 4+/5 to allow return to full participation in ADL, reaching, driving, work, and recreational activities
3. Nonadhered, mobile scar
4. Pain 0/10 to allow her to return to her prior level of function
5. DASH score < 25%
6. Independence in all ADL
7. Independence in home management
8. Driving without limitations
9. Working without limitations
10. Mild recreational activities in 8 weeks with anticipated full return in 12 weeks

Interventions: Skilled services needed for mobilizing (R) shoulder and elbow while protecting healing fracture, education on proper hygiene/self-care while wearing the sling, and appropriate progression of activity for injury protection. She will be treated on outpatient basis 2 to 3 times per week for 8 weeks using therapeutic exercises to restore ROM and normalize soft tissue length, modalities to decrease pain, and soft tissue mobilization for scar adherence. The patient will be progressed to more aggressive activities as able and cleared by referring physician in order to restore function and strength. She will be provided with a home exercise program.

The patient is in agreement with this plan.

Jane Smith, PT

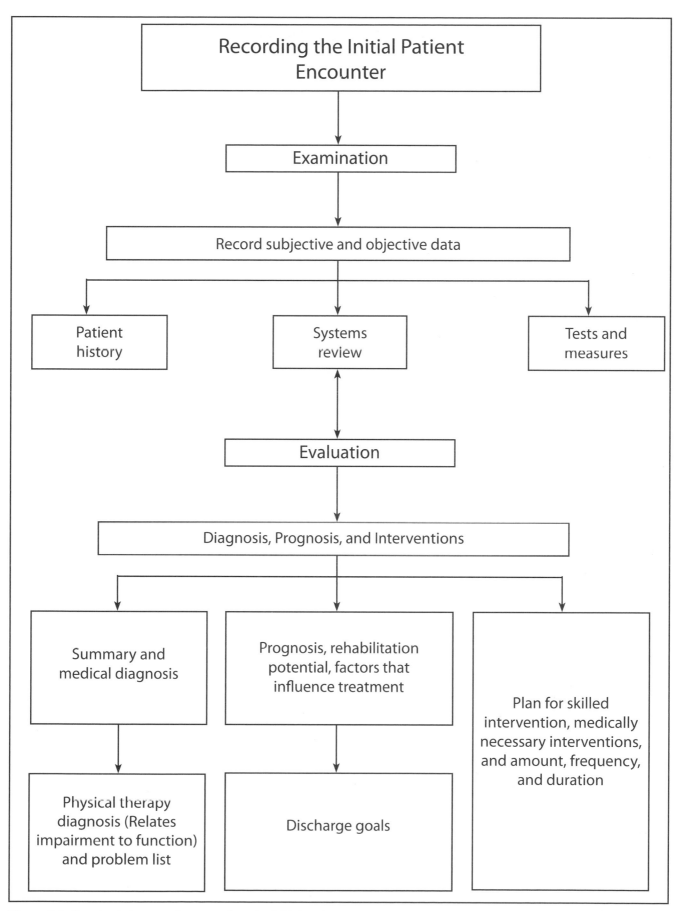

Figure 4-1. Required elements for recording the initial patient encounter.

The Patient's Prognosis

In this part of the documentation, the PT documents the patient's potential for improvement, or rehabilitation potential, as well as any factors that may influence improvement or the interventions (medical, cognitive, psychological, social, economic, etc). These are known as comorbidities, complexities, or complicating factors and they are important so that anyone reading the documentation could understand the reason why progress may be slower than normal.

This section also contains specific, objective, measurable goals that provide a predicted level of improvement with a set time frame for achievement. Goals serve as a PT's measuring stick for monitoring patient progress and determining the effectiveness of the intervention. These are typically written as discharge or outcome goals and reflect what the therapist thinks the patient will be able to do at the end of the episode of care. They may be referred to as long-term goals (LTGs). Goals also reflect the ultimate discharge plan (ie, return to work, return to prior level of function, discharge to long-term care facility, discharge to inpatient rehabilitation facility, etc). As a rule of thumb, there should be a goal for every problem identified in the problem list.

Short-term goals (STGs) may also be included. These are stepping stones toward the final discharge goals and are written in a manner to reflect an associated discharge goal. See the following example:

> *Discharge goal 1: The patient will be independent with ambulating within the community without an assistive device in 8 weeks.*
> A corresponding initial STG could be
> *STG: The patient will be able to ambulate 100' with a straight cane on level surfaces in 4 weeks.*

The Intervention Plan

The PT documents planned interventions that are aimed specifically at the impairments, activity limitations, and participation restrictions identified in the examination. It is this section where the PT describes why his or her unique skills are needed. One documents the procedural items in a statement or list (eg, modalities, exercises, manual therapy, functional training, etc) and provides a *reason* for all interventions in order to demonstrate medical necessity.

Documentation of the intervention plan is comprehensive and includes both procedural and nonprocedural medically necessary activities that will be used to bring about the desired outcome documented in the goals. The nonprocedural items include things such as patient or family education and any coordination, communication, or collaboration with other health care providers. This may also include plans for referral to another health care provider (eg, occupational or speech therapist, orthopedic surgeon, family medicine physician) or setting (eg, outpatient therapy, home health therapy). Finally, one includes the expected amount (times per day), frequency

(times per week), and duration (total length of the episode of care) of services. Example 4-1 provides a sample of documentation completed following an initial encounter with a patient.

DOCUMENTING SUBSEQUENT PATIENT ENCOUNTERS

Interim Notes

As the physical therapy interventions are initiated, the PT documents the patient's care and progress in interim notes. Interim notes include treatment or daily notes, progress notes, reassessments, and reevaluations. The most basic interim note is the treatment note, or daily note. In general, treatment notes serve as records of intervention(s) provided and serve as records to support what was billed or charged to the patient on a given date. They may also include patient data, the patient's response(s) to the interventions in terms of impairments and function, and changes (or need for changes) to the intervention(s) along with an explanation as to why the changes are medically necessary.[4]

CMS provides criteria for treatment notes for physical therapy delivered to Medicare beneficiaries in an outpatient setting. The treatment note "is not required to document medical necessity or appropriateness of the ongoing therapy services."[2(p185)] *At minimum*, the treatment note includes the following[2]:

- Date of treatment
- Identification of each procedure/modality provided and billed, for both timed and untimed codes (see Chapter 12), in language that can be compared with the billing on the claim to verify correct coding
- Total timed code treatment minutes
- Total treatment time in minutes (excluding time for services NOT billable)
- Signature and professional designation of the qualified professional who furnished or supervised the services and a list of persons who contributed (see Appendix C for a template of a treatment note)

Again, this is a specific requirement for documenting services provided to Medicare beneficiaries receiving treatment in an outpatient setting.

Ongoing Assessments and Reevaluations

Throughout the episode of care, one documents changes in the patient's status. After the initial examination and evaluation, there are 3 types of reassessment. First, there is ongoing, regular assessment of patient subjective and objective data that can highlight any changes in the patient's status. This briefer reassessment is a normal part of therapy and can occur each visit or, at minimum, on a weekly basis. These are recorded in the daily notes or, if using CMS terminology, treatment notes.

The second type of assessment is a formal reassessment. Data collection is more comprehensive than what is seen with the regular ongoing assessments that occur more frequently. Formal reassessment includes gathering subjective and objective data similar to that collected on the initial visit to determine whether the patient is making progress toward his or her stated goals. The PTs use these more formal reassessments to determine if the intervention is still medically necessary and to justify ongoing services. These more formal reassessments are documented in progress reports or progress notes. More formal reassessments are generally performed at least every 30 days, but this may vary depending on the setting and the payer (see "Timing Interim Notes").

Like with treatment notes, CMS provides specific criteria for progress notes written in an outpatient setting. The regulations state, "The progress report provides justification for the medical necessity of treatment."[2(p182)] Content requirements for progress reports include the following[2(p185–187)]:

- Dates of treatment interval (current date and date of last or initial exam/evaluation)

- Date the report is written if different from above

- Signature and professional designation of the PT who wrote the report

- Objective report of the patient's relevant subjective comments

- Objective measurements including a description of changes in status; these should be related to current treatment goals

- Documentation of any progress toward or changes in goals:

    - Document if an STG has been met and record new STGs with reference to the corresponding discharge/outcome goal

    Example:

    Discharge goal 1: The patient will be independent with ambulating within the community without an assistive device in 8 weeks.

    STG 1a: The patient will be able to ambulate 100' with a straight cane on level surfaces in 4 weeks (Goal Met)

    New STG 1b: The patient will ambulate 250' without an assistive device on level surfaces in 4 weeks.

    - Document changes to existing discharge/outcome goals

    Example:

    Discharge goal 2 in current plan deleted.

    - Functional documentation. . . including the specific nonpayable G-code and severity modifier (see Chapter 12)

- An overall assessment of progress, or lack thereof

- Plans and justification for continuing treatment given the following:

    - The patient's condition has the potential to improve.

- Maximum improvement is yet to be attained.

- The expectation is that maximum improvement will occur within a reasonable and generally predictable amount of time (see Appendix C for a template of a progress report).

The third type of assessment is a reevaluation. A reevaluation is even more formal and thorough than a reassessment. Reevaluations occur when there are *significant* changes in the patient's status. For example, a PT is seeing a patient in his home and the patient becomes ill, requiring hospitalization. When the patient returns home and the PT resumes treatment, a reevaluation may be warranted. Reevaluation is a separately billable service and there are well-established guidelines as to how frequently they are allowed. The state's practice act or third-party payer guidelines often dictate how frequently a reevaluation can be billed.

After any reassessment or reevaluation, the PT uses his or her clinical judgment to determine whether the current plan of care should be continued or changed. Changing the plan of care requires justification documented in a summary statement by calling the reader's attention to data suggesting a need for change. Any of the following aspects of the plan of care can be changed at any point in the episode of care: the patient's goals; comorbidities, complexities, or complicating factors; rehabilitation potential; procedural and nonprocedural interventions; frequency, amount, or duration of services; or ultimate discharge plan.

Timing Interim Notes

In some physical therapy settings such as outpatient clinics, acute-care hospitals, school settings, and home health, interim notes are written for each visit or encounter the PT or PTA has with a patient. However, in other settings, such as inpatient rehabilitation and skilled nursing facilities, interim notes may be written on a weekly basis, summarizing the patient's status and progress toward goals. State practice acts, payer guidelines, and facility policies dictate the frequency of documentation in various physical therapy settings as well as the timing of reassessments, reevaluations, and completion of progress reports.

Currently, for Medicare beneficiaries being treated in an outpatient setting, treatment notes are required for each visit and a progress report is written at least once every 10 visits.[2] In home health, reassessments and progress reports are also required every 30 days or by the 14th visit. Should services go beyond 14 visits, there should be another reassessment by the 20th visit.[6] In the inpatient rehabilitation setting, progress reports are written on a weekly basis so that the therapist can attend an interdisciplinary conference with other providers to discuss the patient's status toward the established goals. Documentation guidelines for other settings are continuously being added or updated. As a practicing clinician, you will need to continually stay up to date in these requirements. One way to stay current with the CMS regulations is to check periodically on the CMS Web site (www.cms.gov) and specific chapters in the Medicare Benefit Policy Manual, Internet Only Manuals, such as Chapter 1 (inpatient hospitals),[7] Chapter 7 (home health),[6] Chapter 8 (skilled nursing),[8] Chapter 12 (comprehensive outpatient rehabilitation facilities),[9] and Chapter 15 (outpatient facilities).[2]

Discharge Notes

The *Guide to Physical Therapist Practice* defines discharge as ending services provided in a single episode of care when goals and outcomes have been achieved.[1] When the patient is being discharged from physical therapy, the PT performs a discharge assessment and records the data in a discharge note, or summary, to provide a record of the patient's final subjective and objective status. The PT compares and summarizes initial and discharge data so that the medical record reflects changes in the patient's status achieved through the episode of care. The PT may also describe how the intervention(s) helped in bringing about patient change. In the discharge summary, the PT documents the patient's progress toward the established goals (met, not met, ongoing) and any plans for continuing care elsewhere, including formal physical therapy or through an independent home exercise program.[4]

The *Guide to Physical Therapist Practice* differentiates discharge from discontinuation.[1] Discontinuation is defined as the process of ending services provided in an episode of care when the patient: (1) declines, or refuses further intervention; (2) is unable to participate, as in cases when there is a significant change in the medical condition or there is a change in financial or psychosocial resources allowing the patient to continue; or (3) will no longer benefit.[1] Nevertheless, clinically, the term discharge is most often used to denote ending the episode of care, regardless of the reason. More information on discharge notes is provided in Chapter 11.

THE PHYSICAL THERAPY ASSISTANT AND INTERIM NOTES

It is the sole responsibility of the PT to write the evaluative portions of the initial documentation, assessments, reevaluations, and discharge notes. This includes all elements of the initial plan of care such as the prognosis, diagnosis, and interventions as well as any changes within or to an existing plan of care. The state's physical therapy practice act determines what the PTA can legally document. In most cases, the assistant may write subjective patient comments and collect and record objective data after performing tests and measures delegated by the PT. Additionally, the assistant can add comments that reflect changes in subjective or objective data from previous visits, or encounters. For example, a PTA has been working with Mr. Smith for the last 3 treatments for gait training after a total knee arthroplasty. On day 1 of treatment, the patient ambulated 50 feet with minimal assist for balance and verbal cues for sequencing the lower extremities and the assistive device. On treatment day 3, the patient ambulated 150 feet requiring close supervision. The assistant may call attention to these specific changes in status documenting:

Ambulation improved from 50' with minimal assist required for balance and verbal cues for sequencing to 150' with supervision.

The PTA can also, in most states, document plans for future treatment as long as they are consistent with, or fall within, the most recent plan of care written by the PT.

REVIEW QUESTIONS

1. Differentiate the *examination* process from the *evaluation* process according to the Patient/Client Management Model. Examination- recording objective/subjective patient data evaluation- using this information to form a diagnosis/prognosis

2. In a clinical setting and according to CMS, examination and evaluation are referred to as _____. "the initial evaluation"

3. Subjective data are taken from patient, family, or caregiver

4. List 5 examples of subjective data. history of present illness, mechanism of injury, date of injury, prior medical history, chief complaints

5. Following collection of subjective data (history taking), the PT should perform
   (a) _____ and
   (b) _____.

6. The results of (a) and (b) above are considered _____ data.

7. During the examination, the physical therapist measures impairment, _____, and participation _____.

8. Give 2 reasons for documenting impairment and function.

9. The evaluation process guides the physical therapist in determining and documenting the _____, _____, and _____.

10. The "summary" of the patient provided in the assessment portion of the note should serve to link _____ and _____.

11. Factors such as a secondary medical diagnosis that adversely influence treatment are known as _____.

12. Goals written on the initial documentation are _____ goals, or _____ goals.

13. Differentiate between a treatment note and a progress note, according to CMS.

14. What information must be included in the progress note that is not required to be in the treatment note?

15. How are STGs related to outcome or discharge goals?

16. Differentiate between regular assessments, reassessments, and reevaluations.

17. In what settings are progress notes written on a weekly basis rather than for each encounter?

18. A PT can bill separately for a _____ , as opposed to a regular assessment, which is expected and not separately billable.

19. List 5 things found in a discharge summary.

20. How does the *Guide to Physical Therapist Practice* differentiate discharge from discontinuation?

APPLICATION EXERCISES

1. List 10 common tests and measures used by PTs. Differentiate those that measure impairments from those that measure function.

2. Create an outline that could serve as a template for each of the following types of documentation:
   a. The initial documentation
   b. Treatment/daily note
   c. Progress note/report (completed following a reassessment)
   d. Discharge note

3. Look at the following interventions. For each, write a sentence as to how you could show medical necessity for that intervention.
   a. Lower extremity strengthening
      Example:
      Lower extremity strengthening will be used to increase independence and safety with sit to stand and ambulation.
   b. Balance training
   c. Gait training
   d. Transfer training
   e. Trunk rotation range of motion
   f. Sensory reeducation
   g. Electrical stimulation
   h. Ultrasound
   i. Cross-friction massage
   j. Manual lymph drainage

4. Look at the following initial examination and evaluation note. Identify the following:
   a. Three pieces of subjective data
   b. Three pieces of objective data
   c. The patient summary and medical diagnosis
   d. The PT diagnosis or description of how impairments are leading to functional problems
   e. Specific problems to be addressed
   f. Comorbidities
   g. Potential for improvement
   h. Outcome goals
   i. An explanation of the need for skilled services
   j. Referral to another provider
   k. List of medically necessary interventions
   l. Frequency, amount, and duration of services
   m. Ultimate plan for discharge
   n. Informed consent

This patient was admitted to an inpatient rehabilitation unit 4 days after transtibial amputation.

Patient Name: Robert Houston

Date: January 15, 2013

Problem: 72 y.o. male s/p (R) standard transtibial amputation 1/11/13. Referred for evaluation for inpatient rehabilitation stay and treatment of amputation. PMH includes NIDOM, COPD, PVD, and HTN. Current meds include glucophage, albuterol, salmeterol, and atenolol.

Subjective: Patient history: Long history of chronic wounds on the right foot with recent development of osteomyelitis and gangrene; underwent transtibial amputation 1/11/13. Pt. is a nonsmoker and nondrinker, although smoked 1 pack per day for 30 years. Quit when he was 50 y.o.

C/C: Phantom pain from the right foot that can get to 8/10, unable to "get around," and decreased endurance.

L/S: Patient is retired coal miner. Reports his height at 6' 2" and weight at 225#. He lives alone in single-level house, with 2 steps at the entrance and no handrail. States he has never used an assistive device. Has been independent with all ADL and IADL prior to admission. Reports that he drove and played occasional golf. Has one son living about 2 hours away who can assist on the weekends.

Patient goals: Return to independent living, active lifestyle, including driving. Wants to obtain a prosthetic device.

Objective: Systems review: CP system: HR 92 bpm, BP 135/88, RR 12. Integumentary system: Sutures present along anterior aspect of the distal tibia. Musculoskeletal system: Impaired. See below. Neuromuscular system: Impaired. See below. Communication/cognition: Not impaired.

Tests and measures: Capillary refill: (L) foot is intact. Sensation: Decreased sensation to light touch around the scar on residual limb and on the (L) foot (Intact to 5.09 monofilament). Incision: Distal residual limb 5" horizontal incision, minimal red bloody drainage, no tension, complete closure, sutures intact, no s/s of infection AROM: (R) hip flexion 90°, extension 0°, abduction 40°, adduction 10°, knee flexion 60°, knee extension –10°. (L) hip flexion 120°, extension 0°, abduction 40°, adduction 10°, knee flexion 140°, knee extension 0°. PROM: Right hip flexion 95°, knee extension –5°, knee flexion 65°. Strength: (B) UEs and left LE are 5/5 throughout; Right LE not assessed because of surgery. Pulses: Popliteal artery 2+ bilaterally. Balance: Not impaired when standing in parallel bars. Anthropometrics: Residual limb length is 7" from medial joint line.

Girth	Right	Left
Knee joint	52 cm	50 cm
2" below	52.5 cm	40 cm

<u>Endurance</u>: Unable to ambulate more than 25' without shortness of breath. During mobility RPE was 12.

<u>Functional assessment</u>: <u>Bed mobility</u>: Independent rolling and scooting. <u>Transfers</u>: Supine ↔ sit with minimal assist × 1; sit ↔ stand with minimal assist × 1; toilet transfers performed with minimal assist × 1. <u>Gait</u>: Ambulated 10' × 1 in parallel bars with contact guard assist × 1 and 25' with standard walker with minimal assist × because of to poor endurance and fatiguing quickly. Also needed assist because of impaired balance with walker. <u>Wheelchair management</u>: Requires maximal assist for wheelchair parts management; propels ~20' on level surfaces and then requires a rest break. <u>Interventions for 1/15/13</u>: 20 minutes of exercises including hip AROM: flexion, extension, abduction, and adduction; knee flexion and extension; hamstring stretching; and towel propping.

Assessment: 72 y.o. male 4 days s/p transtibial amputation with decreased ROM, strength, endurance, and balance resulting in impaired mobility including transfers and functional ambulation. PT diagnosis: Impaired motor function, muscle performance, range of motion, gait, locomotion, and balance associated with amputation. Patient is not safe to return home at this time and requires inpatient stay for improving safety to live alone.

Problems to be addressed with PT:

<u>Impairments</u>:

1. Decreased ROM (R) LE
2. Decreased strength (R) LE
3. Decreased sensation
4. Edema
5. Incision present
6. Impaired balance with walker
7. Phantom pain
8. Impaired endurance

<u>Functional limitations</u>:

1. Decreased independence with ambulation
2. Decreased independence with transfers
3. At risk for nonhealing incision and skin abnormalities
4. Unable to drive
5. Unable to perform necessary IADL (grocery shopping, going to bank, etc)

6. Wants to return to active lifestyle using a prosthetic device

<u>Prognosis</u>: Good for established goals (below) although complexities such as COPD, PVD, HTN, and impaired endurance and decreased sensation on the (L) LE may slow progress.

<u>Discharge goals</u>: After 3 weeks, the patient will:

1. Demonstrate full A/PROM in the right LE with no contractures—necessary for normal prosthetic ambulation
2. Demonstrate right LE strength 4/5 also to allow normal prosthetic ambulation
3. Be independent with skin care and monitoring skin on the residual limb and (L) LE
4. Ambulate 200' with walker with prosthesis and least restrictive assistive device to allow independence with home ambulation
5. Transfer in/out of bed and sit to/from stand independently
6. Participate in a community outing with only minimal assist × 1
7. Return home independently and obtain appropriate home modifications and equipment

Plan: Patient to receive skilled services for improving functional mobility including gait and transfer training because of amputation and decreased endurance and balance. Requiring education on mobility, skin care, and preparing residual limb for prosthesis.

See pt. for 1 hour bid for ~3 weeks for intensive rehabilitation to work on achieving the above goals through active and passive exercise to increase limb mobility to maximize use of prosthesis, strengthening to allow normal prosthetic gait, endurance training to improve mobility, gait, and transfer training, pain modulation for phantom pain, balance activities to improve safety. Patient will also require consultation with prosthetist. The patient is motivated and agrees with the above plan.

Jane Smith, PT

References

1. American Physical Therapy Association. The *Guide to Physical Therapist Practice*. 2nd ed. Alexandria, VA: APTA; 2003.
2. Centers for Medicare & Medicaid Services. Covered medical and other health services. *Medicare Benefit Policy Manual*. Publication 100-02. http://www.cms.gov/Regulations-and-Guidance/Guidance/Manuals/Downloads/bp102c15.pdf. Accessed May 16, 2012.
3. American Physical Therapy Association. Guidelines: Physical therapy documentation of patient/client management. http://www.apta.org/uploadedFiles/APTAorg/About_Us/Policies/BOD/Practice/DocumentationPatientClientMgmt.pdf. Accessed May 16, 2012.
4. Hebert LA. Basics of Medicare documentation for physical therapy. *Clinical Management in Physical Therapy*. 1981;1(3):13-14.
5. American Physical Therapy Association. Defensible documentation. http://www.apta.org/Documentation/Defensible Documentation/. Accessed May 16, 2012.

6. Centers for Medicare & Medicaid Services. Medicare Benefit Policy Manual Publication No. 100-02 Ch. 7. Available at: http://www.cms.gov/Regulations-and-Guidance/Guidance/Manuals/Downloads/bp102c07.pdf. Accessed May 16, 2012.

7. Centers for Medicare & Medicaid Services. Inpatient hospital services covered under part A. *Medicare Benefit Policy Manual.* Publication 100-02. http://www.cms.gov/Regulations-and-Guidance/Guidance/Manuals/Downloads/bp102c01.pdf. Accessed May 16, 2012.

8. Centers for Medicare & Medicaid Services. Coverage of extended care (SNF) services under hospital insurance. *Medicare Benefit Policy Manual.* Publication 100-02. http://www.cms.gov/Regulations-and-Guidance/Guidance/Manuals/Downloads/bp102c08.pdf. Accessed May 16, 2012.

9. Centers for Medicare & Medicaid Services. Comprehensive outpatient rehabilitation facility (CORF) coverage. *Medicare Benefit Policy Manual.* Publication 100-02. http://www.cms.gov/Regulations-and-Guidance/Guidance/Manuals/Downloads/bp102c12.pdf. Accessed May 16, 2012.

Chapter 5

Documentation Formats

Mia L. Erickson, PT, EdD, CHT, ATC

CHAPTER OUTLINE

Documentation Formats
  Narrative Notes
  Problem-Oriented Medical Record ✗
  Subjective, Objective, Assessment, and Plan Notes
  Functional Outcomes Report ✗
Contemporary Approach
Templates and Forms
Dictation
The Electronic Medical Record

CHAPTER OBJECTIVES

Upon completion of this chapter, the reader will be able to:
1. Compare and contrast narrative notes, problem-oriented medical records, SOAP notes, and functional outcomes reports.
2. Describe the problem-status-plan documentation format.
3. Differentiate between information found in the S, O, A, and P portions of a SOAP note.
4. Explain the rationale for blending functional information into SOAP.
5. Organize patient information using the different documentation formats.
6. Describe the current legislation regarding electronic medical records and electronic health records.
7. Differentiate between the electronic medical records and electronic health records.
8. Identify positive and negative aspects of electronic medical records.

Erickson ML, Utzman RR, McKnight R. *Physical Therapy Documentation:*
From Examination to Outcome, Second Edition (pp 41-63).
© 2014 SLACK Incorporated.

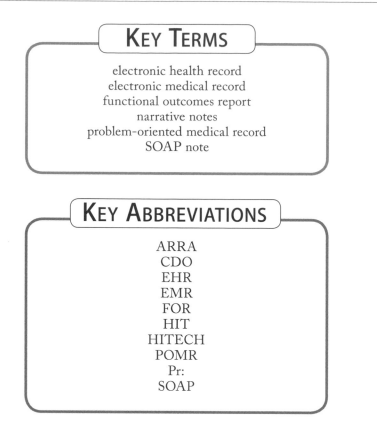

DOCUMENTATION FORMATS

Documentation in physical therapy practice can take on a variety of formats, and the format you use will depend on the type of patients being treated, the practice setting, state laws and practice acts, reimbursement requirements, and the type of patient encounter. It will also depend on whether you are using paper-based documentation or an electronic medical record. Traditional documentation formats include narrative reports, problem-oriented medical records (POMR), SOAP notes, and the functional outcomes reports (FOR). A more contemporary approach, however, includes a combination of these. This "combined" approach is discussed in the latter part of this chapter.

Narrative Notes

In narrative documentation, the clinician describes the patient encounter with pertinent information provided in paragraph format. The narrative format can be used when documenting initial patient encounters (Example 5-1A), interim notes (Example 5-1B), reevaluations (Example 5-1C), and discharge summaries (Example 5-1D). Besides typical patient care documentation, there are other times when the narrative format is the most appropriate to use. Narrative notes are sometimes the easiest to use when you just need to describe the details of a situation and you are trying to paint a vivid description of what happened. Examples include describing a sequence of events,

brief interactions with patients, conversations with other health care providers, or any other situation that requires a detailed explanation and no other documentation formats are appropriate (Example 5-1E).

Authors have identified several problems with the narrative record. First, because of the lack of structure, there is potential for the writer to omit important details. This can be a problem because it is assumed that if it is not documented, it did not happen. The lack of structure combined with a high degree of variability among clinicians writing in this format make narrative notes difficult to read and necessary information difficult to locate.[1] For example, it would be very time consuming for a case manager to sort through a chart filled with unstructured narrative entries to locate information regarding the patient's ability to transfer. Following the clinician's problem-solving process can also be difficult in narrative reports.[2] Quinn and Gordon[1] recommended developing an outline, or template, of necessary information to include so that important details about the patient or the treatment session are not inadvertently omitted. One may also use headings to denote different sections or different types of data. Headings give the narrative note structure, making it more readable and allowing someone to find information in the note more quickly. Headings often used are shown in Table 5-1.

Problem-Oriented Medical Record

Lawrence Weed[2] developed the POMR in the 1960s. Weed indicated that narrative documentation was confusing and unorganized, making it difficult to use.

Example 5-1A. Initial Documentation: Narrative Format

very detailed but very difficult to find the info you need quickly

Physical Therapy

Initial Examination and Plan of Care

Patient: John Smith

Date of Service: January 3, 2012 11:15

Reason for Referral: Evaluate and treat for (L) elbow pain

Physician: Dr. Jones

Chart Number: 346254

Mr. Smith is a 35 y.o. man with (L) elbow pain. Pt. reports developing pain after spending the weekend painting his house 3 months ago. The pt. reports using ice and taking meds (OTC ibuprofen) initially but this didn't help. Saw his physician for a yearly physical and mentioned the elbow pain. His physician suggested "trying a few weeks of PT." Chief complaint at this time is pain (6/10 at worst and 2/10 at best) that increases with heavy grip, computer use, and using hand tools. Denies temperature changes and numbness. Has not had any X-rays or imaging procedures. Pt. denies history of a similar problem or prior elbow pain. Reports overall health is good with no relevant medical or surgical history. Pt. lives alone and works as an accountant. Reports primary functional deficits including painful work-related activities, home management tasks, and recreational activities such as mountain biking and kayaking. Global functional rating is 85 out of 100. The patient's goals for therapy include pain reduction allowing him to participate in functional and recreational tasks and prevention of recurrence.

Review of systems: Review of systems revealed BP, 120/84; HR, 78 bpm; and RR, 12. Neurological and integumentary systems are not impaired. No impairments in cognitive or communicative status. There is palpable point tenderness on the (L) lateral epicondyle and wrist extensor origin. AROM of (R) UE is WNL (elbow 0/145 degrees); (L) shoulder, wrist, and hand are WNL; (L) elbow is −10/140 degrees; c/o pain at end range elbow flexion, extension, forearm supination, and wrist extension; cervical A/PROM also WNL and pain free. PROM of the (L) elbow is 0/145 with normal end feel but c/o pain. MMT indicates 5/5 strength throughout (B) UE except (L) wrist extension and supination are 4/5 with pain. All special provocation tests for (L) elbow are unremarkable except a (+) tennis elbow test. Pain-free grip strength (R) 100, 110, 108# (L) 65, 60, 55# with pain. (−) edema compared bil. Neurovascular structures are intact. Sensation is WNL compared bil. DASH functional assessment score 28/100 (see attached). Treatment today consisted of: 1) Education: Instruction in HEP, activity modification including grip and activities to avoid, instruction in safe use of tennis elbow strap; 2) pulsed 1 MHz US @ 50% duty cycle 1.5 w/cm^2 × 8 min to (L) lateral epicondyle; 3) wrist extensor stretching with neutral and UD wrist, cross-friction massage to extensor origin. Total exam time 30 min and total tx time 20 min.

Assessment and plan (plan of care): 35 y.o. LHD male with medical dx of (L) lateral epicondylitis (3-month history) and PT dx: Impaired mobility, function, muscle performance, and ROM due to connective tissue dysfunction (practice pattern 4D). Pain and decreased ROM are limiting the patient's ability to perform functional grip and complete necessary home and recreational activities. Specific problems include: elbow pain and tenderness; decreased AROM (L) elbow; (L) wrist, and elbow weakness; decreased grip strength; painful work-related, home management, and recreational tasks; limited in carrying heavy objects and opening/closing jars. Pt. has good potential for improvement but may require extended time because of chronic nature of his condition. Expected LTGs to be met by 3/3/12: A) Decrease pain 90-100%; B) A/PROM (L) elbow WNL and pain free; C) 5/5 strength (L) without pain; D) Pain-free grip strength = (R); E) Pain-free work-related, home management, and recreational tasks; F) No difficulty in carrying heavy objects or opening/closing jars; G) DASH score decreased < 10%. STGs to be met in 2 wks: A-1) Decrease pain 10-20%; B-1) Increase A/PROM by 5 degrees for flexion and extension; C-1) Strength 4+/5; D-1) Increase pain-free grip strength 10-15#; E-1) Decrease pain during work-related, home management, and recreational tasks by 50%; F-1) Mild difficulty (per DASH) in carrying heavy objects or opening/closing jars; G-1) DASH score decreased 10-15%. Skilled services needed to administer modalities and friction massage to soften adhesions associated with chronic inflammation and decrease pain; will also teach pt. safe stretching program to increase flexibility and eccentric strengthening for appropriate connective tissue elongation; and will instruct in activity modification. PT intervention will be provided 2 to 3×/wk × 6 to 8 wks. This pt. is in agreement with the plan of care.

Sue Smith, DPT

Good for: documenting something out of the ordinary

Example 5-1B. Interim Note: Narrative Format

PT Interim Note

Patient: John Smith

Date of Service: January 6, 2012 11:30

Reason for Referral: Evaluate and treat for (L) elbow pain

Physician: Dr. Jones

Chart Number: 346254

Pt. reports pain at level 6/10 at worst and 0 to 1/10 at best. Pain still increases with heavy grip, computer use, using hand tools. Reports compliance with HEP. No adverse effects from last tx. Palpable point tenderness on (L) lateral epicondyle and wrist extensor origin. AROM of (L) elbow is −10/140 degrees. Treatment today consisted of: 1) pulsed 1 MHz US @ 50% duty cycle 1.5 w/cm^2 × 8 min to (L) lateral epicondyle; 2) wrist extensor stretching with neutral and UD wrist, cross-friction massage to extensor origin; 3) reviewed pt.'s HEP; and 4) ice massage × 5 min to (L) extensor origin (total tx time 20 min). Pt. notes slight improvement in pain since last visit. No other changes in objective or subjective data. Continue with current plan of care.

Sue Smith, DPT

Example 5-1C. Reassessment: Narrative Format

PT Reassessment and Progress Report

Patient: John Smith

Date of Service: January 30, 2012 12:00

Reason for Referral: Evaluate and treat for (L) elbow pain

Physician: Dr. Jones

Chart Number: 346254

Pt. has been receiving PT since 1/3/12 for (L) lateral epicondylitis. Chief complaint at this time is still pain (3/10 at worst and 0/10 at best). It continues to increase with heavy grip and using hand tools. No longer having pain during work-related activities. Reports primary functional deficits at this time including painful home management tasks and recreational activities. Global functional rating is 90 out of 100. The patient's present therapy goals include returning to prior level of activity without pain and regaining all ROM. Musculoskeletal system shows palpable point tenderness on the (L) lateral epicondyle and wrist extensor origin. AROM of (L) elbow is −5/145 degrees with minimal to no pain at end range elbow flexion, extension, forearm supination, or wrist extension. MMT indicates (L) wrist extension and supination are 4+/5 with pain upon extension only. Continues to have (+) tennis elbow test. Pain-free grip strength (R) 100, 110, 108#; (L) 85, 90, and 87#. DASH functional assessment score 13/100 (see attached). Treatment today consisted of: 1) wrist extensor stretching with neutral and UD wrist, cross-friction massage to extensor origin, eccentric strengthening to wrist extensors. Total re-exam time 30 min and tx time 30 min.

Assessment and plan (plan of care): Pt. has made progress with his therapy program. Worst pain has decreased from 6/10 to 3/10; pain during ADL has decreased, and global rating of function has increased 5%. DASH functional assessment has also decreased 15%, which suggests significant change. Continues to show s/s of (L) lateral epicondylitis. PT dx: impaired mobility, function, muscle performance, and ROM due to connective tissue dysfunction (practice pattern 4D). Pain with gripping continues to limit his home management tasks and participation in recreational activities. Specific problems include: elbow pain and tenderness, decreased AROM (L) elbow, muscle weakness, decreased grip strength, painful home management and recreational tasks, limited in carrying heavy objects, and opening/closing jars. Pt. continues to show good potential for improvement but may require extended time because of chronicity. Expected LTGs to be met by 3/3/12: A) Decrease pain 90-100%; B) A/PROM (L) elbow WNL and pain free; C) 5/5 strength (L) without pain; D) Pain-free grip strength = (R); E) pain-free work-related, home management, and recreational tasks; F) no difficulty in carrying heavy objects or opening/closing

(continued)

Example 5-1C. Reassessment: Narrative Format, continued

jars; G) DASH score decreased < 10%. STGs set at initial visit: A-1) Decrease pain 10-20% (Goal met); B-1) Increase A/PROM by 5 degrees for flexion and extension (Goal met); C-1) Strength 4+/5 (Goal met); D-1) Increase pain-free grip strength 10-15# (Goal met); E-1) Decrease pain during work-related, home-management, and recreational tasks by 50% (Goal met); F-1) Mild difficulty (per DASH) in carrying heavy objects or opening/closing jars (Goal met); G-1) DASH score decreased 10-15% (Goal met). For the next 2 weeks, we will continue to work toward meeting the above stated LTGs; seeing the pt. 1-2×/wk. Skilled services are needed to administer friction massage and teach pt. safe exercise progression so that his symptoms do not increase. Tx will include: continued stretching, eccentric strengthening, modalities if needed, and progression to return to normal activities. This pt. is in agreement with the new plan of care.

Sue Smith, DPT

Example 5-1D. Discharge Summary: Narrative Format

Discharge Summary

Patient: John Smith

Date of Service: March 1, 2012 11:30

Reason for Referral: Evaluate and treat for (L) elbow pain

Physician: Dr. Jones

Chart Number: 346254

Dates of PT Services: January 3 through March 1, 2012 (12 visits)

Pt. has been receiving PT for (L) lateral epicondylitis since 1/3/12. At present pain is 0/10 and occasionally goes to 1-2/10 with heavy activities like using hand tools. No pain with normal ADL, home management, recreation, community, or work activities. Denies activity limitations or participation restrictions. Global functional rating is 98/100. He reports that he can perform his HEP without difficulty and the "stretching has helped." Negative palpable point tenderness; AROM (L) elbow 0/145 degrees; wrist extension and supination strength are 5/5 and pain free; (–) tennis elbow test; Pain-free grip strength (R) 100, 110, 110# and (L) 98, 105, 100#; DASH functional score 8/100 (8%). Pt. has made good progress including improving AROM, MMT, and grip strength to normal. Also has shown reduced pain (90-100%) and improved function during normal ADL, home management, work, community, and recreational activities (initial DASH score 28/100, current 8/100). All LTGs have been met. Plan to d/c PT at this time to (I) HEP. Pt. will RTC if further problems arise.

Sue Smith, DPT

Example 5-1E. Other Narrative Examples

Inpatient Setting:

02/09/12: Went to see pt. for gait and transfer training. Pt. lying in bed and reported feeling sick. Refused PT today.

05/03/12: Attempted to see pt. this afternoon. Spoke with nursing staff prior to session; they indicated that pt. was to receive a blood transfusion and asked to withhold PT today. Will attempt to see pt. in the morning if cleared.

Outpatient Setting:

04/05/12: Pt. called this morning reporting that she was not improving with therapy. Stated that she planned to call her physician. Canceled appointment for today. Will call to reschedule if needed.

04/05/12: Saw pt. today for follow-up visit after fabrication and fitting of (L) WHFO wrist cock-up orthosis. Remolded edge around thenar eminence and at MCP crease to allow more thumb and finger motion and decrease skin pressure at distal palmar crease. Pt. indicated improved motion with decreased pain after adjustment. Will have pt. return if needed for further orthosis adjustments.

Jon Smith, PT

Table 5-1

Common Headings Used to Add Structure to Documentation

Patient's name	Muscle tone
Medical record number	Endurance
Date of service	Balance
Reason for referral	Integumentary
History of present illness or problem	Sensation
Mechanism of injury	Functional assessment
Chief complaint(s)	Interventions provided
Medications	Mobility
Imaging procedures	Gait
Prior and current functional status	Transfers
General health	Summary
Prior or past medical history	Medical diagnosis
Pain intensity or pain rating	PT diagnosis
Lifestyle or living situation	Problem list
Screening/systems review/review of systems	Rehab potential
Observation	Complicating factors
Palpation	Short-term goals
Range of motion	Long-term goals
Strength	Planned interventions

The POMR provided structure to the medical record by organizing patient information and treatment according to the patient's problems. The first page of the medical record included the patient's problem list, and this served as the "table of contents" for the remainder of the medical record (Example 5-2A). Subsequent entries, or interim notes, included subjective and objective clinical data, an overall impression (Imp:), treatment or therapy (Tx: or Rx:), and a future plan for each problem (Example 5-2B).

Major advantages of the POMR have been reported.[3-7] It provided organization and structure to the medical information and included a comprehensive list of the patient's problems. It allowed the reader to quickly identify care provided and future management plans for each problem, thereby making documentation more problem oriented, or problem centered. The POMR also allowed a clinician interested in a particular problem to go directly to that aspect of the note, thus easing communication among care providers. Finally, the POMR provided a chronological sequence of interventions for a particular problem, better outlining the problem-solving process.

Regardless of the benefits to the structure provided with the POMR, authors have reported problems with it as well. First, it was difficult for providers to see the "whole patient" because of the way it is organized by individual patient problems.[5] For example, in more complex cases, it was possible that a clinician working with breathing might not be aware of postural problems without reading separate chart entries. Yet, reading all chart entries for each problem was very time consuming. In addition, for patients with multiple problems, the POMR became increasingly complex, requiring an extraordinary amount of time for an individual managing multiple problems.

In the mid-1970s, several authors reported on the use of the POMR in rehabilitation.[3,4,7-9] Reinstein et al[9] supplemented the POMR with information specific to rehabilitation. Later they reported this form of documentation did improve communication among team members in the rehabilitation setting, but it was far too difficult for complicated patients often encountered.[7]

A more recent problem-oriented approach, although it did not necessarily evolve from the POMR, is the problem-status-plan approach. In this format, one documents the patient's functional problem, his or her current functional status, the day's addressing of the problem interventions, and the rehabilitative plans to address the problem. In this approach, one may also integrate the goal for the particular functional problem. Using this approach, the reader is able to identify the problem for which each intervention is directed. This approach is often used in interim notes for early intervention and school-based settings and can be useful for parents. It is also being integrated into electronic documentation templates (Table 5-2).

Subjective, Objective, Assessment, and Plan Notes

SOAP is an acronym for **S**ubjective, **O**bjective, **A**ssessment, and **P**lan. The SOAP format evolved from the POMR initially described by Weed[2] and also provided structure to medical record entries. Unlike the POMR, one SOAP note, as it is often called, includes information pertaining to all of the patient's problems. In physical therapy, the SOAP note became a stand-alone format for documentation used for initial documentation (Example 5-3A),

Example 5-2A. Initial Documentation: POMR Format

Physical Therapy

Initial Examination and Plan of Care

Patient: John Smith

Date of Service: January 3, 2012

Reason for Referral: Evaluate and treat for (L) elbow pain

Physician: Dr. Jones

Chart Number: 346254

Problem list:

1. Elbow pain and tenderness
2. Decreased AROM (L) elbow
3. Muscle weakness
4. Decreased grip strength
5. Painful work-related, home management, and recreational tasks
6. Limited in carrying heavy objects and opening/closing jars

Subjective: Medical dx: (L) lateral epicondylitis; referred to PT by Dr. Jones

HPI: 35 y.o. LHD man reports developing pain after spending the weekend painting his house 3 months ago. The pt. reports using ice and taking meds (OTC ibuprofen) initially but this didn't help. Saw his physician for a yearly physical and mentioned the elbow pain. His MD suggested "trying a few weeks of PT." Reports that he has not had any X-rays or imaging procedures. Pt. denies hx of a similar problem or prior elbow pain.

C/C: Pain (6/10 at worst and 2/10 at best) that increases with heavy grip, computer use, using hand tools. Denies temperature changes and numbness. Reports primary functional deficits including painful work-related activities, home management tasks, and recreational activities such as mountain biking and kayaking. Global functional rating is 85% out of 100.

PMH: Reports overall health is good with no relevant medical or surgical history.

Lifestyle: Pt. lives alone and works as an accountant.

Pt.'s goals: Pain reduction to allow improvement in functional tasks and prevention of recurrence.

Objective: Systems review: BP, 120/84; HR, 78 bpm; and RR, 12. Neurological and integumentary systems are not impaired. No impairments in cognitive or communicative status.

Pain: Musculoskeletal system shows palpable point tenderness on the (L) lateral epicondyle and wrist extensor origin.

AROM: (R) UE is WNL (elbow 0/145 degrees); (L) shoulder, wrist, and hand are WNL except elbow is −10/140; c/o pain at end range elbow flexion, extension, forearm supination, and wrist extension; cervical A/PROM also WNL and pain free.

PROM: (L) elbow is 0/145 with normal end feel but c/o pain.

Strength: MMT indicates 5/5 strength throughout (B) UE except (L) wrist extension and supination are 4/5 with pain.

All special provocation tests for (L) elbow are unremarkable except a (+) tennis elbow test. Pain-free grip strength (R) 100, 110, 108#; (L) 65, 60, 55# with pain.

Anthropometric measurements: (−) edema compared bil.

Neurovascular: Neurovascular structures are intact. Sensation is WNL compared bil. Function: DASH functional assessment score 28/100 (see attached).

Time: Exam: 30 min

Imp: Pain, ROM loss, and weakness are limiting the patient's ability to grip, carry heavy objects, open/close lids, perform full home management duties, and participate in normal work tasks. PT dx: impaired mobility, function, muscle performance, and ROM due to connective tissue dysfunction (Practice Pattern 4D). Pt. has good potential for improvement but may require extended time because of chronicity.

Expected LTGs: to be met by 03/03/12: A) Decrease pain 90-100%; B) A/PROM (L) elbow WNL and pain free; C) 5/5 strength (L) without pain; D) Pain-free grip strength = (R); E) Pain-free work-related, home management, and recreational tasks; F) No difficulty in carrying heavy objects or opening/closing jars; G) DASH score < 10%.

STGs to be met in 2 wks: A-1) Decrease pain 10-20%; B-1) Increase A/PROM by 5 degrees for flexion and extension; C-1) Strength 4+/5; D-1) Increase pain-free grip strength 10-15#; E-1) Decrease pain during work-related, home management, and recreational tasks by 50%; F-1) Mild difficulty (per DASH) in carrying heavy objects or opening/closing jars; G-1) DASH score decreased 10-15%.

Tx today: 1) Education: HEP, activity modification to decrease tight fisting and overuse activities, discussed activities to avoid and modify handle grips, proper use of tennis elbow strap; 2) pulsed 1 MHz US @ 50% duty cycle 1.5 w/cm^2 × 8 min to (L) lateral epicondyle, wrist extensor stretching with neutral and UD wrist, cross-friction massage to extensor origin. Tx time: 20 min

Plan: Skilled services are needed to administer modalities and friction massage to soften adhesions associated with chronic inflammation and teach pt. safe stretching program to increase flexibility, eccentric strengthening for appropriate connective tissue elongation, and activity modification. PT interventions will be provided 2-3×/wk × 6-8 wks. This pt. is in agreement with the plan of care.

Sue Smith, DPT

Example 5-2B. Interim Note: POMR Format

A separate entry for each problem is completed; therefore, for this date of service, there would be potentially 6 entries in the chart. Two entries are provided as examples using this format.

Patient: John Smith
Date of Service: January 3, 2012 11:30
Reason for Referral: Evaluate and treat for (L) elbow pain
Physician: Dr. Jones
Chart Number: 346254

Problem List:

1. Elbow pain and tenderness
2. Decreased AROM (L) elbow
3. Muscle weakness
4. Decreased grip strength
5. Painful work-related, home management, and recreational tasks
6. Limited in carrying heavy objects and opening/closing jars

Note for Problem #1: Elbow pain and tenderness

S: Pt. reports pain at level 6/10 at worst and 0 to 1/10 at best. Pain still increases with heavy grip, computer use, using hand tools. Reports compliance with HEP.
O: Palpable point tenderness on (L) lateral epicondyle and wrist extensor origin. Treatment today consisted of: 1) pulsed 1 MHz US @ 50% duty cycle 1.5 w/cm^2 × 8 min to (L) lateral epicondyle; 2) reviewed pt.'s HEP; and 3) Ice massage × 5 min to (L) extensor origin. (Total tx time 20 min).
Imp.: Pt. notes slight improvement in pain since last visit as evidenced by decrease in pain. No other changes in objective or subjective data.
Plan: Continue with current plan of care.

Note for Problem #2: Decreased AROM (L) elbow

S: No subjective comments on ROM
O: AROM of (L) elbow is −10/140 degrees. Treatment today consisted of: 1) wrist extensor stretching with neutral and UD wrist, cross friction massage to extensor origin
Imp.: No changes in ROM since initial visit.
Plan: Continue with current plan of care.

Sue Smith, DPT

Table 5-2

Hypothetical Note Using Problem-Status-Plan Approach

Problem	Current Status	Intervention	Plan
1. Dependent sit to stand transfers	Transfers sit to stand with mod ⓐ × 1	15' ther ex including bridging, mini-squats, quad strengthening	Progress LE strengthening program
2. Unable to ambulate independently in the home because of fall risk	Timed up-and-go score 13 s; ambulates 150' with cane and supervision	15' balance activities with verbal assist for upright posture and trunk support	Progress balance program with assist for safety
3. Unable to perform community ambulation	Uses w/c with assist from wife for community mobility	15' gait training to increase gait velocity, independence, and safety	Progress gait training as patient's safety increases

Example 5-3A. Initial Examination and Evaluation: SOAP Format

Physical Therapy

Initial Examination and Plan of Care
Patient: John Smith
Date of Service: January 3, 2012
Physician: Dr. Jones
Chart Number: 346254

Pr: <u>Reason for referral</u>: Evaluate and treat for (L) elbow pain; <u>Medical diagnosis</u>: (L) lateral epicondylitis

S: <u>HPI</u>: 35 y.o. LHD man reports developing pain after spending the weekend painting his house 3 months ago. The pt. reports using ice and taking meds (OTC ibuprofen) initially but this didn't help. Saw his physician for a yearly physical and mentioned the elbow pain. His physician suggested "trying a few weeks of PT." Has not had any X-rays or imaging procedures. Pt. denies history of a similar problem and prior elbow pain.

<u>C/C</u>: Pain (6/10 at worst and 2/10 at best) that increases with heavy grip, computer use, using hand tools. Denies temperature changes and numbness. Reports primary functional deficits include painful work-related activities, home management tasks, and recreational activities such as mountain biking and kayaking. Global functional rating is 85 out of 100.

<u>PMH</u>: Reports overall health is good with no relevant medical or surgical history.

<u>L/S</u>: Pt. lives alone and works as an accountant.

<u>Patient's goals</u>: Pain reduction allowing improvement in functional tasks and prevention of recurrence.

O: <u>Systems review</u>: BP, 120/84; HR, 78 bpm; RR, 12. Neurological and integumentary systems: not impaired. Cognitive or communicative status: not impaired. Impairments noted in musculoskeletal system, see below.

<u>Pain</u>: Musculoskeletal system shows palpable point tenderness on the (L) lateral epicondyle and wrist extensor origin.

<u>AROM</u>: (R) UE is WNL (elbow 0/145 degrees); (L) shoulder, wrist, and hand are WNL except elbow is −10/140; c/o pain at end range elbow flexion, extension, forearm supination, and wrist extension; cervical A/PROM also WNL and pain free.

<u>PROM</u>: (L) elbow is 0/145 with normal end feel but c/o pain.

<u>Strength</u>: MMT indicates 5/5 strength throughout (B) UE except (L) wrist extension and supination are 4/5 with pain. All special provocation tests for (L) elbow are unremarkable except a (+) tennis elbow test. Pain free grip strength (R) 100, 110, 108# (L) 65, 60, 55# with pain.

<u>Anthropometric measurements</u>: (−) edema compared bil.

<u>Neurovascular</u>: Neurovascular structures are intact. Sensation is WNL compared bil.

<u>Function</u>: DASH functional assessment score 28/100 (see attached).

<u>Tx today</u>: 1) Education: HEP, activity modification, use of tennis elbow strap; and 2) pulsed 1 MHz US @ 50% duty cycle 1.5 w/cm^2 × 8 min to (L) lateral epicondyle, wrist extensor stretching with neutral and UD wrist, cross friction massage to extensor origin. <u>Time</u>: Exam: 30 min; Treatment: 20 min; Total: 50 min.

A: 35 y.o. LHD male with medical dx of (L) lateral epicondylitis (3 month history) and PT dx: impaired mobility, function, muscle performance, and ROM due to connective tissue dysfunction (practice pattern 4D). Pain and decreased ROM are limiting the patient's ability to perform functional grip and complete necessary home and recreational activities.

<u>Problem list</u>: Elbow pain and tenderness; decreased AROM (L) elbow; (L) wrist and elbow weakness; decreased grip strength; painful work-related, home management, and recreational tasks; limited in carrying heavy objects and opening/closing jars.

<u>Rehab potential</u>: Good potential for improvement but may require extended time because of chronic nature of his condition.

<u>Expected LTGs</u>: to be met by 3/3/12:

A) Decrease pain 90-100% to allow improved function such as grip

B) A/PROM (L) elbow WNL and pain free

C) 5/5 strength (L) without pain

D) Pain-free grip strength equal to the (R)

E) Pain-free work-related, home management, and recreational tasks

F) No difficulty in carrying heavy objects or opening/closing jars

G) DASH score decreased to < 10%

<u>STGs</u>: to be met in 2 wks:

A-1) Decrease pain 10-20%

B-1) Increase A/PROM by 5 degrees for flexion and extension

C-1) Strength 4+/5

D-1) Increase pain-free grip strength 10-15#

E-1) Decrease pain during work-related, home management, and recreational tasks by 50%

(continued)

Example 5-3A. Initial Examination and Evaluation: SOAP Format, continued

F-1) Mild difficulty (per DASH) in carrying heavy objects or opening/closing jars

G-1) DASH score decreased 10-15%

P: <u>Skilled services</u>: Needed to administer modalities and friction massage to soften adhesions associated with chronic inflammation and decrease pain; will also teach pt. safe stretching program to increase flexibility and eccentric strengthening for appropriate connective tissue elongation; and will instruct in activity modification. PT intervention will be provided 2-3×/wk × 6-8 wks. This pt. is in agreement with the plan of care.

Sue Smith, DPT

Example 5-3B. Interim Note: SOAP Format

PT Interim Note

Patient: John Smith
Date of Service: January 6, 2012 11:30
Physician: Dr. Jones
Chart Number: 346254

Pr: <u>Reason for referral</u>: Evaluate and treat for (L) elbow pain

S: Pt. reports pain at level 6/10 at worst and 0 to 1/10 at best. Pain still increases with heavy grip, computer use, using hand tools. Reports compliance with HEP. No adverse effects from last tx.

O: Palpable point tenderness on (L) lateral epicondyle and wrist extensor origin. <u>AROM</u>: (L) elbow is −10/140 degrees. <u>Treatment today</u>: 1) pulsed 1 MHz US @ 50% duty cycle 1.5 w/cm^2 × 8 min to (L) lateral epicondyle; 2) wrist extensor stretching with neutral and UD wrist, cross-friction massage to extensor origin; 3) reviewed patient's HEP; and 4) ice massage × 5 min to (L) extensor origin. (Total tx time 20 min).

A: Pt. notes slight improvement in pain since last visit (0-1/10 versus 2/10). No other changes in objective or subjective data.

P: Continue with current plan of care.

Sue Smith, DPT

Example 5-3C. Reassessment: SOAP Format

PT Reassessment and Progress Report

Patient: John Smith
Date of Service: January 30, 2012 (Visit #12) 12:00
Physician: Dr. Jones
Chart Number: 346254

Pr: <u>Reason for referral</u>: Evaluate and treat for (L) elbow pain; <u>Medical diagnosis</u>: (L) lateral epicondylitis

S: <u>C/C</u>: pain (3/10 at worst and 0/10 at best). It continues to increase with heavy grip and using hand tools. No longer having pain during work-related activities. <u>Functional status</u>: Reporting primary functional deficits at this time including painful home management tasks and recreational activities. Global functional rating is 90 out of 100.

<u>Patient's goals</u>: Present therapy goals include returning to prior level of activity without pain and regaining all ROM.

O: Musculoskeletal system shows palpable point tenderness on the (L) lateral epicondyle and wrist extensor origin. <u>AROM</u>: (L) elbow −5/145 degrees with minimal to no pain at end range elbow flexion, extension, forearm supination, or wrist extension.

<u>Strength</u>: (L) wrist extension and supination are 4+/5 and pain with extension only, (+) tennis elbow test. Pain-free grip strength (R) 100, 110, 108#; (L) 85, 90, and 87#.

<u>Functional assessment</u>: DASH functional assessment score 13/100 (see attached). <u>Today's tx</u>: 1) wrist extensor

(continued)

Example 5-3C. Reassessment: SOAP Format, continued

stretching with neutral and UD wrist, cross friction massage to extensor origin, eccentric strengthening to wrist extensors. Total re-exam time 30 min and tx time 30 min.

A: Pt. has made progress with his therapy program. Worst pain has decreased from 6/10 to 3/10, pain during ADL has decreased, and global rating of function has increased 5%. DASH functional assessment has also decreased 15%, which suggests significant change. Continues to show s/s of (L) lateral epicondylitis. Pain with gripping continues to limit his home management tasks and participation in recreational activities.

PT dx: Impaired mobility, function, muscle performance, and ROM due to connective tissue dysfunction (practice pattern 4D).

Problem list: Elbow pain and tenderness; decreased AROM (L) elbow; muscle weakness; decreased grip strength; painful home management and recreational tasks; limited in carrying heavy objects; and opening/closing jars.

Rehab potential: Pt. continues to show good potential for improvement but may require extended time because of chronicity.

Expected LTGs to be met by 3/3/12:

A) Decrease pain 90-100% to allow improved function such as grip

B) A/PROM (L) elbow WNL and pain free

C) 5/5 strength (L) without pain

D) Pain-free grip strength = (R)

E) Pain-free work-related, home management, and recreational tasks

F) No difficulty in carrying heavy objects or opening/closing jars

G) DASH score decreased to < 10%

STGs from initial evaluation:

A-1) Decrease pain 10-20% (Goal met)

B-1) Increase A/PROM by 5 degrees for flexion and extension (Goal met)

C-1) Strength 4+/5 (Goal met)

D-1) Increase pain-free grip strength 10-15# (Goal met)

E-1) Decrease pain during work-related, home management, and recreational tasks by 50% (Goal met)

F-1) Mild difficulty (per DASH) in carrying heavy objects or opening/closing jars (Goal met)

G-1) DASH score decreased 10-15% (Goal met)

P: For the next 2 weeks, we will continue to work toward meeting the above-stated LTGs seeing the pt. 1-2x/wk. Skilled services are needed to administer friction massage and teach pt. safe exercise progression so that his symptoms do not increase. Tx will include: continued stretching, eccentric strengthening, modalities if needed, and progression to return to normal activities. This pt. is in agreement with the new plan of care.

Sue Smith, DPT

Example 5-3D. Discharge Summary: SOAP Format

Discharge Summary

Patient: John Smith

Date of Service: March 1, 2012 12:00

Physician: Dr. Jones

Chart Number: 346254

Dates of PT Services: January 3 through March 1, 2012 (12 visits)

Pr: Reason for referral: Evaluate and treat for (L) elbow pain; Medical diagnosis: (L) lateral epicondylitis

S: C/C: At present pain is 0/10 and occasionally goes to 1–2/10 with heavy activities like using hand tools. No pain with normal ADL, home management, recreation, community, or work activities. Denies activity limitations or participation restrictions. Global functional rating is 98/100. He reports that he can perform his HEP without difficulty and the "stretching has helped."

O: Pain: Negative palpable point tenderness; AROM: (L) elbow 0/145 degrees; Strength: wrist extension and supination strength are 5/5 and pain free; (–) tennis elbow test;

pain-free grip strength (R) 100, 110, 110# and (L) 98, 105, 100#; Function: DASH functional score 8/100 (8%).

A: Pt. has made good progress including improving AROM, MMT, and grip strength to normal. Also has shown reduced pain (90-100%) and improved function during normal ADL, home management, work, community, and recreational activities (initial DASH score 28/100, current 8/100). LTGs: All have been met.

P: d/c PT at this time to (I) HEP. Pt. will RTC if further problems arise.

Sue Smith, DPT

return to clinic

Figure 5-1. Subjective data included in the "S" or Subjective section of the SOAP note.

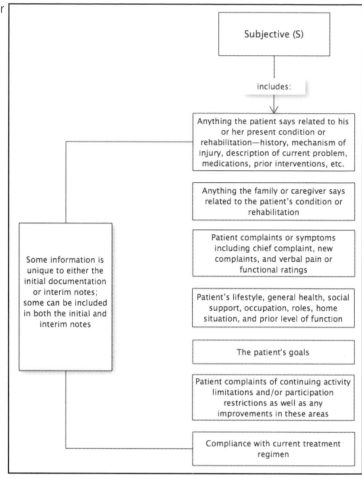

interim notes (Example 5-3B), reevaluations (Example 5-3C), and discharge summaries (Example 5-3D). The S, or subjective section, includes anything the patient tells you pertaining to his or her injury, disease, condition, or illness. The subjective section also includes any information provided by the patient's family or caregivers. The O, or objective, section includes relevant tests and measures, the patient's functional status, and physical therapy interventions performed for that day of service. The A, or assessment, includes the interpretation, or impression, and the P stands for plan. It includes any plans for managing the patient and his or her physical therapy problems. Specific information provided in the S, O, A, and P portions of the notes can be found in Figures 5-1 through 5-4. A "Problem" (Pr:) section may precede the SOAP note. When used, the Problem section contains information pertaining to the medical diagnosis, the physical therapy referral, and information from the medical record (see Example 5-3A). There is more about the Problem and specific SOAP contents in subsequent chapters.

Although SOAP notes provide a consistent, concise format for documenting the patient's subjective remarks, objective exam findings, the provider's overall impression, and the plan of care, it, too, is often challenged. Historically, the subjective section has centered on the patient's complaints, primarily pain. Second, objective findings were written in terms of impairments, such as range of motion, strength, and balance. Assessments were written in terms of how the patient tolerated the treatment (eg, "The patient tolerated the treatment well.") and the plan was often written very generally (eg, "Continue per plan."). Furthermore, the relationship between improvements in the patient's impairments and improved functional capabilities were usually implied or assumed, rather than described in specific detail with reference to objective data.[10,11] Additionally, the relationship between interventions and improvement was also implied rather than explained. These problems resulted in documentation centered on the patient's complaints and impairments rather than progress toward functional restoration. More recent and even bigger issues with the SOAP format are the tendency to leave out (1) the description of the skill used by the clinician providing the services and (2) the discussion of why treatment is medically necessary. Both these are required for more contemporary documentation.

Nevertheless, the SOAP format is widely used by a variety of medical and rehabilitation professionals, and its components—S, O, A, and P—are well-known in medical record documentation. The SOAP format can be an appropriate form of documentation but the contents need

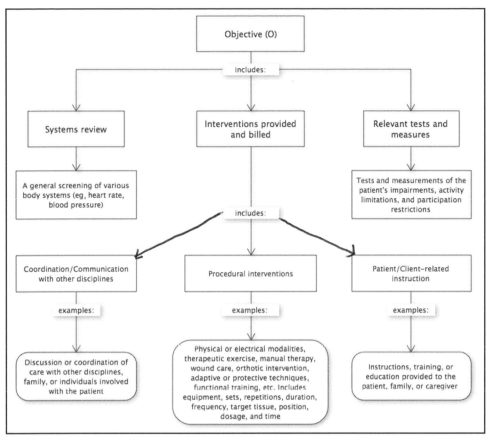

Figure 5-2. Objective data included in the "O" or Objective section of the SOAP note.

to include more contemporary concepts such as disablement, function, medical necessity, and need for skilled care. It must also be written to show logical decision making by using subjective and objective information to support the assessment and plan.

Functional Outcomes Report

The FOR is another documentation format used in rehabilitation. Quinn and Gordon[1] describe the FOR as a type of documentation that focuses on the patient's ability to perform meaningful functional activities rather than isolated impairments. Advantages of the FOR have been identified. In using the FOR, the writer emphasizes the relationship between the patient's impairments and his or her activity limitations and participation restrictions. Using functional terminology helps improve readability for non–health care providers reviewing documentation.[1,12]

Regardless of positive and negative aspects of the different documentation formats, the SOAP format is generally the most common documentation format used in physical therapy practice. Nearly 2 decades ago, Abeln[12] suggested making the following additions to SOAP in order to integrate more functional concepts:

1. Subjective (S) section: Describe the functional problems as stated by the patient

2. Objective (O) section: Assess and objectively measure the patient's functional status, including functional activities that are specific to that patient

3. Assessment (A) section:
   a. List only those impairments being addressed with therapy
   b. Describe how improvement in impairments will lead to improvement in function limitations
   c. Provide complicating factors, such as comorbidities
   d. Write goals using functional terminology

Since then, the trend for integrating function has increased. Examples 5-3A through 5-3D are written in a manner to show integration of functional concepts into the SOAP structure.

CONTEMPORARY APPROACH

This chapter outlines several different formats to document patient/client management. In clinical practice, you are likely to encounter a wide variety of documentation formats, but it is important that you adhere to your facility's approved format, the state's practice act, federal regulations, and payer requirements. Additionally, there

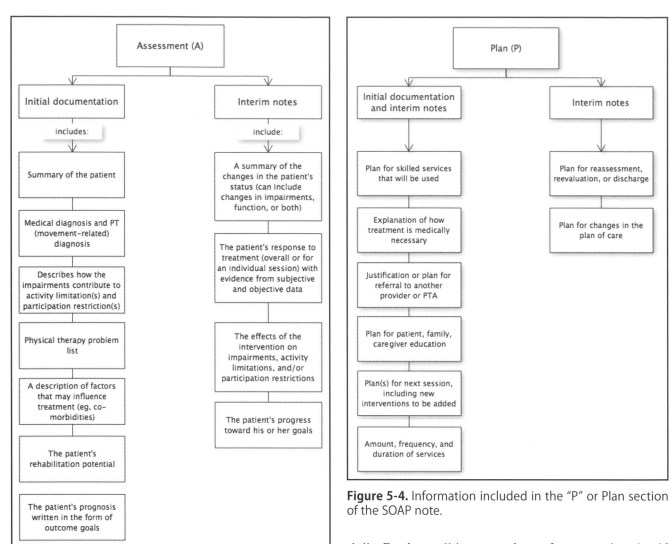

Figure 5-3. Information included in the "A" or Assessment section of the SOAP note.

Figure 5-4. Information included in the "P" or Plan section of the SOAP note.

should be some general consistency in the documentation format used, although there may be times when another format (eg, narrative) is needed. These reasons have been described. It is the author's experience that the SOAP format continues to be most widely used, but the integration of patient function (like that described in the FOR) is increasingly more common. In addition, there are electronic documentation packages incorporating various aspects of each of the documentation formats, including the problem-status-plan format. Although there is no evidence suggesting superiority of one format over another, you will soon find that in real-world clinical practice, you are likely to apply principles from the different formats; therefore, it is important to be familiar with the different ones available.

The authors of this text have selected the basic SOAP format to provide a framework for learning documentation

skills. Readers will be exposed to information that should go into the S, O, A, and P portions of the note. In addition, readers will be exposed to how aspects of the patient/ client management model can fit into the basic SOAP structure (Table 5-3). The SOAP format was selected because of its prevalence in clinical practice and because of its adaptability to a variety of documentation styles and physical therapy practice settings. It is also a good format for students who are learning basic documentation skills. The authors believe teaching the SOAP format provides learners with the essential knowledge of required components. Once in the clinical setting, the individual can reorganize the components into the clinical setting's format, transferring what they have learned about the traditional SOAP structure into the setting's format. Well-written clinical documentation, however, does not depend on the format being used; the key to quality documentation is the content. Well-written records include pertinent subjective and objective data and justify a reasonable, medically necessary, and skilled plan of care. Well-written records are necessary for physical therapy practice and, therefore, quality and content are emphasized.

		Table 5-3	
		Components of the Patient/Client Management Model and Their Location in the Initial Documentation Using the SOAP Format	
Patient/Client Management	*Includes*	*What to Record*	*Location in the SOAP Note*
Examination	1. History	• Subjective data	S, or Subjective section

	2. Systems review: Cardiovascular system Integumentary system Musculoskeletal system Neuromuscular system Cognitive/communicative ability	• Objective data
		  • Results of systems review
		  • Results of tests and measures
			O, or Objective section

	3. Tests and measures		
Evaluation	Clinical judgment, problem-solving process, determining PT diagnosis, prognosis, and the plan of care	• Brief summary of the patient, synthesizing exam findings, including relationship between impairments and function • PT diagnosis (can use ICD-9 or a practice pattern from the *Guide to Physical Therapist Practice*) • PT problem list • Factors influencing treatment (eg, comorbidities) • Rehab potential • Prognosis written by the PT in form of discharge goals.	A, or Assessment section
		• Summarizes need/plans for skilled services Need/plans for referral to another health care provider*	A or P
		• Planned interventions and rationale to give medical necessity • Frequency, duration, and amount of treatment • Any ultimate plans	P, or Plan section

*These items may be written in the A or P sections of a SOAP note depending on the PT's judgment. In this text these items appear in the P section.

Data compiled from American Physical Therapy Association. Defensible documentation. http://www.apta.org/AM/Template.cfm?Section=Home&NAVMENUID=2505&CONTENTID=37071&DIRECTLISTCOMBOIND=D&TEMPLATE=/MembersOnly.cfm. Accessed July 30, 2007.

TEMPLATES AND FORMS

Templates and fill-in forms (either paper or electronic) are frequently used by health care organizations in order to facilitate documentation. Utilization of templates and forms can ease the documentation burden; improve speed, efficiency, and productivity; and minimize writing. Well-designed templates and forms can facilitate accuracy, prompt clinicians to provide necessary data, improve consistency in documentation across patients and providers, and help meet documentation guidelines set forth by third-party payers. Templates or fill-in forms can be used for initial documentation, interim notes, reevaluations, discharge summaries, and progress letters written to physicians. Several examples have been provided in Appendix C. The *Guide to Physical Therapist Practice*[13] and Defensible Documentation[14] also include documentation templates for use in physical therapy practice.

Templates and forms also provide a mechanism for multidisciplinary documentation in which each discipline has its own section to complete on the same form. In some settings, federal regulations require use of specialized forms. For example, Medicare requires the Minimum Data Set (MDS; version 3.0 was the version used at the time of writing this text) in skilled nursing facilities,[15] the Inpatient Rehabilitation Facility Patient Assessment Instrument (IRF PAI) in inpatient rehabilitation hospitals,[16] and the Outcome and Assessment Information Set (OASIS) in home health.[17] The Individuals with Disabilities in Education Act (IDEA)—a federal law that governs states to provide a free appropriate public education for all children with disabilities residing in the state between birth and age 21 years—requires therapists in early intervention and school-based programs to complete special kinds of multidisciplinary documentation.[18] Therapists working in early intervention programs (birth to age 3 years) complete documentation known as an Individualized Family Service Plan (IFSP)—a model of which can be found at http://idea.ed.gov/part-c/search/new. Therapists working in a school-based setting complete an Individualized Education Plan (IEP).[19]

Clinical, or critical, pathways are another type of multidisciplinary documentation done in settings where providers treat a high volume of certain patient types. These are useful when there are specific goals or expectations for each day of service following a specific surgery or procedure (eg, out of bed, transfer, ambulate, stairs) and there are multiple service providers (eg, nursing, physical therapy, nutrition) (Table 5-4).

A disadvantage of templates and forms is that, if not carefully designed, a form may not allow for complete documentation of all pertinent information.[20] A mechanism to include any pertinent patient information should exist. For example, there should be a section that allows documentation of unique aspects of the treatment encounter not provided on the standard template. It is important that the therapist not be constrained by limits of a form. This is true for students who might feel as though they cannot deviate from the form. Additionally, templates and forms are often geared toward the patient population treated most at the facility and it might be difficult to use these forms when documenting care provided to patients with less common diagnoses.

DICTATION

Dictation is verbal communication of information that is transcribed by an individual or computer software into written documentation. Transcription occurs either immediately as the therapist speaks or at a later time from a recording. Dictation and transcription offer the benefit of flexibility, allowing the clinician to include any pertinent information within the documentation. Although facilities using dictation and transcription usually subscribe to a generalized structure for documentation (eg, the SOAP format), flexibility is allowed within that structure. Dictation can be a time-saver once a clinician becomes familiar with the activity because it takes less time to speak information than to write it. An additional benefit of dictation and transcription is the documentation's readability. This leads to a reduction of error in clinical practice due to the inability to read the health care provider's handwriting. Drawbacks of dictation include the cost, hardware, typographical errors, and the error due to the transcriptionist's inability to accurately hear or understand the clinician's voice—although digital recorders are improving in this area.

When dictating, it is important for the clinician to speak clearly and include any details that need to be included in the final document. In this instance, care must be taken to clearly describe how the final transcription should appear. For example, the clinician will need to verbalize if the information needs to be in a table format or when there is a new heading. Once transcription is complete, the clinician reads all dictated notes for errors. Errors should be corrected on the original form in the same manner as all error correction for patient care documentation.

THE ELECTRONIC MEDICAL RECORD

Computerized documentation is one of the fastest growing areas of health care and information technology industries. This trend has been facilitated by several national initiatives.[21,22] In February 2009, President Obama signed the American Recovery and Reinvestment Act (ARRA). This legislation includes the Health Information Technology for Economic and Clinical Health Act (HITECH),[23] which provides incentives to health care providers who demonstrate "meaningful use" of certified electronic medical records (EMR).

"Meaningful use" rules are developed by the DHHS and include 3 stages. Stage 1 includes criteria for the amount and type of information (eg, patient demographics, height, weight, lab values) recorded in an EMR,[24] and stages 2 and

Table 5-4
Hypothetical Clinical Pathway for Patient Post-Total Hip Arthroplasty

Postoperative Day	Mobility (PT)	Exercise (PT)	Self-care (OT)	Precautions (PT/OT)
1 Date: _7/7/12_	AM treatment: Transferred supine to sit and bed to w/c with mod ⓐ ×1 for weight bearing and safety. Sit to stand with min ⓐ ×1. Patient ambulated in parallel bars PWB 50% with min ⓐ ×1 for verbal instructions and safety because of light-headedness. PM treatment: Patient ambulated 20' with standard walker with min ⓐ ×1 for verbal cueing for weight-bearing precautions and safety because of light-headedness.*	Patient instructed in bedside exercises bid. Performed 25 reps: 1. Ankle pumps 2. Quadriceps isometrics 3. Hip abduction 4. Heel slides 5. Gluteal isometrics		Provided patient with hip precautions; patient verbalized understanding
Goal	Out of bed to PT Department Ambulates 15–25' (50% weight bearing) with minimal to moderate assist ×1	Bedside exercises per protocol to increase ROM and circulation	Self-hygiene at sink with minimal assistance	Hip precautions provided
	Goal met	Goal met		Goal met
Additional note in chart?	Yes __✓__ No _____		Yes _____ No _____	
Treatment time	28'	10'		2'
Signature	Susan Smith, DPT	Susan Smith, DPT		Susan Smith, DPT
2 Date: _7/8/12_	AM treatment: Transferred supine to sit and bed to w/c with min ⓐ ×1 for maintaining hip precautions and safety. Sit to stand with min ⓐ ×1. Patient ambulated 50' with standard walker with CGA ×1 for verbal cueing for reminders for weight-bearing precautions and sequencing gait pattern PM treatment: Same as am	Patient instructed in bedside exercises bid. Performed 25 reps: 1. Ankle pumps 2. Quadriceps isometrics 3. Hip abduction 4. Heel slides 5. Gluteal isometrics		Patient able to verbally provide hip precautions with minimal prompts
Goal(s)	Out of bed to PT department Ambulates 25–50' (50% weight bearing) with minimal to moderate assist ×1	Exercises in PT department to increase ROM and circulation	Self-hygiene at sink performed with verbal cues	Hip precautions reviewed
	Goal met	Goal met		Goal met
Additional note in chart?	Yes __✓__ No _____		Yes _____ No _____	
Treatment time	28'	10'		2'
Signature	Susan Smith, DPT	Susan Smith, DPT		Susan Smith, DPT

Italicized text indicates documentation completed by the PT.

Figure 5-5. Sample electronic documentation.

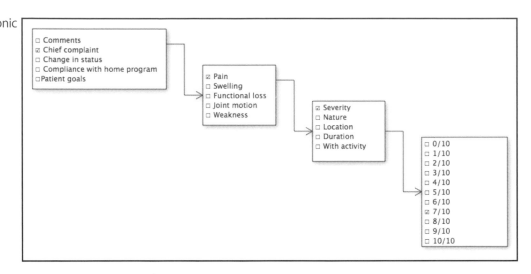

3 are expected to include information related to information exchange, including a process for easily sharing patient information (eg, lab results and patient summaries). As of 2012, both Medicare and Medicaid were implementing incentive programs for those implementing the electronic record.[25] Importantly, in 2015, Medicare-eligible professionals, hospitals, and critical access hospitals that do not demonstrate meaningful use of a certified electronic system will have payment adjustments or penalties in their Medicare reimbursement.[25]

The terms *electronic medical record* (EMR) and *electronic health record* (EHR) are often used interchangeably; however, they are different concepts.[26] The EMR is defined as "an application environment composed of the clinical data repository, clinical decision support, controlled medical vocabulary, order entry, computerized provider order entry, pharmacy, and clinical documentation applications. This environment supports the patient's EMR across inpatient and outpatient environments, and is used by health care practitioners to document, monitor, and manage health care delivery within a care delivery organization (CDO)."[26(p2)] The EMR is a legal record of the patient's encounter at a single CDO, or health system, and is owned by the CDO. Patients may have viewable access to their EMR through a portal but the patient cannot interact with the data. The EHR, which is owned by the patient, includes information from various CDOs where the patient has had encounters. It allows the patient full access as well as the ability for the patient to append the information.[26]

A goal of transitioning health care providers to the EMR is to facilitate the development of the nationally integrated EHR system that would allow providers across numerous health systems and in different geographic locations to access a patient's health information. This can be established only if the EMR for individual CDOs are at a "level that can create and support the robust exchange of information between stakeholders within a community or given region."[26(p3)] The ARRA and HITECH legislation provided funds for the Office of the National Coordinator for Health Information Technology, which has set a goal

for the use of an EHR for each person in the United States by 2014 and a nationwide health information technology (HIT) infrastructure that allows for the electronic use and exchange of medical information.[27]

In physical therapy practice, there are various types of recordkeeping systems still being used. In some practices, clinicians continue to use paper and other practices have large integrated, end-to-end computerized systems. An end-to-end EMR is a single platform, or database, that includes various applications such as scheduling, documentation, billing, and data management.[28] These various applications share data, and data entry by an office or administrative employee populates the clinician's data entry portal. Physical therapists working in large health care systems document in the EMR that is part of a larger hospital-based system. The current trend is moving physical therapy providers toward electronic software that integrates several organizational activities.

Electronic documentation software packages in physical therapy often consist of commonly used templates based around body systems or regions that incorporate check boxes, pull-down menus, and other time-saving efforts (Figures 5-5 and 5-6). Software packages contain ways to document a variety of note types including initial documentation, interim notes, progress notes, and discharge summaries. Like with paper templates, the electronic templates are used to standardize terminology and consistency between patients and clinicians and improve communication throughout an organization. Within this standardization, however, a level of flexibility for the needs of various departments can and should be achieved because all patient cases may not fit into the standard template. Documentation software should have flexibility for the development of templates that will match the needs of different settings and patients. Some software packages can generate special types of documentation such as letters, progress reports, and flow sheets populated with previously recorded data with a few clicks and this can be a significant time-saving benefit for clinicians. Other benefits are the ability to track the number of visits and insurance

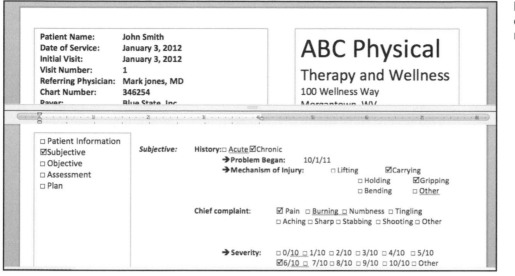

Figure 5-6. Hypothetical creation of an electronic note.

authorization. It also allows the clinicians or office staff to set prompts designed to remind the PT and PTA when various processes need to occur, such as reassessments, plan-of-care updates, and insurance recertification.

Vreeman et al[22] performed a systematic review of the literature to determine the benefits, barriers, and keys for successful implementation of EHRs within physical therapy practice settings. The authors found that published data on the use of an EHR for physical therapy are limited. Upon review of 18 articles that met the author's inclusion criteria, the following benefits of using the EHR were identified: (1) improved reporting capabilities, (2) increased operational efficiency, (3) better interdepartmental communication, (4) improved data accuracy, and (5) improved access to data for future research. Decreased time requirements for electronic data entry rather than hand entry improved data accuracy, resulted in less redundancy, and allowed employees to be more efficient. Improved readability of the electronic record over handwritten information and the ability for multiple users to access information simultaneously improved interdepartmental communication. These benefits in turn helped facilitate improved clinical decision making.[22]

Over the years, the sophistication of documentation software has grown, allowing databases that will provide data for research, monitor productivity, and analyze outcomes data, which all provide benefit to the profession at large. Data collection can occur at a local or individual clinic level or at multiple clinical sites using more integrated systems that are connected through larger networks. APTA's CONNECT,[29] a computerized patient documentation system that allows scheduling, documentation, and some billing procedures, allows transmission of patient data into a national outcomes database. The aggregate data can provide information to PTs, patients, and payers.[29]

Vreeman et al[22] reported barriers to using an EHR. These barriers included (1) the change to workflow or work behavior, (2) the potential for software or hardware inadequacy, and (3) the initial and ongoing need for staff training. However, most of these problems are resolvable over time.[22] Also, it is difficult to articulate medical necessity, need for skilled care, and a description of skilled care provided in an electronic system via check boxes and pull-down menus. This is largely due to the individual patient differences as well as the need for clinicians to create individualized plans of care. So, this information may need to be documented in a free-text field rather than a check box because they are such important components of the documentation. The need to free text a lot of information quickly decreases the system's efficiency. It is also important for clinicians not to get into a routine documenting the same things for every patient; because computerized software generates standard phrases, notes can quickly start appearing the same for each patient. Furthermore, the clinic must be prepared for regularly scheduled system backups, upgrades, and maintenance of computer hardware and software. There must also be processes for storing system backup files so that critical information is not lost. Finally, there must be a mechanism to record, give reason for, and authenticate late entries.[30]

Another consideration is the cost–benefit ratio. Cost consideration not only includes the financial outlay for the software or subscription, hardware, and network but also includes the cost in time associated with staff training and technical support. Subscriptions to Web-based platforms frequently include software technical support, but costs of technical support for the hardware components and network, as well as maintenance and upgrades, must also be considered.

Security and confidentiality are additional considerations and these policies and procedures must be in place. This is especially true for documentation software that

REVIEW QUESTIONS

1. What are the similarities and differences between narrative notes, SOAP notes, POMR, and FOR?

2. What are the advantages and disadvantages of narrative notes, SOAP notes, POMR, and FOR?

3. Give examples of information you would find in the S, O, A, and P sections of the note.

S - medical history, chief complaints   A - diagnosis
O - blood pressure, ROM   P - frequency, duration, treatment plan

4. What is the importance of documenting a patient's functional status?

5. What ways can a patient's functional status be written into a SOAP note?

6. How can disablement be integrated into SOAP documentation?

7. How can elements of the Patient/Client Management Model be integrated into a SOAP note?

8. What is the problem-status-plan note? In what settings is it used?

9. Name the multidisciplinary documentation forms/templates commonly used in skilled nursing units, home health agencies, inpatient rehabilitation hospitals, school systems, and early intervention.

10. Name the positive and negative aspects of the EMR.

APPLICATION EXERCISES

1. Read the following statements and determine if it would belong in the S, O, A, or P sections of a SOAP note.

   a. **O** Gait: Ambulated 50' × 2 WBAT (R) LE with min ⓐ × 1 & verbal cues to advance the (R) LE

   b. **S** Pt. reports HEP has helped increase AROM

   c. **P** Pt. will RTC 2 times per week for 4 weeks

   d. **O** Transfers: bed to/from chair with mod ⓐ × 2; requires stabilization to block the knee and assist to stand

   e. **A** Pt. progressing toward goals set on the initial evaluation

   f. **S** Patient's wife stated that she has been assisting the patient with his HEP

   g. **P** Speak with the physician about decrease in BP upon transferring from supine to sitting position

   h. **O** AROM: (R) knee 0 to 135 degrees

   i. **A** Improvements in knee AROM allow patient to sit without difficulty and ascend/descend stairs with less difficulty

   j. **S** Pt. feels that he is benefiting from the strengthening exercises in that he is now able to open jars and lids (I)

   k. **P** Pt. will be seen for bid gait training

   l. **S** Pt. denies use of assistive device prior to admission

   m. **A O** Gait distance improved from 25' to 150' over the last week

   n. **O A** Demonstrating (L) neglect making her unsafe during gait and transfers

o. **O** Muscle performance: All (R) LE strength is 5/5

p. **O** Vitals: HR, 95 bpm; RR, 12; BP, 140/95

q. **A** Pt. has improved his ability to transfer in/out of bed since initial visit

r. **P** Will contact physician about possible d/c as pt. is no longer benefiting from the interventions

s. **A** Pt.'s endurance is poor because of inactivity

t. **A**
S Pt. c/o inability to brush teeth and eat with (R) hand because of decreased AROM of the (R) elbow

u. **A** Pt. is unable to drive or perform safe community mobility at this time

A v. **O** Edema in (R) ankle has decreased 2 cm

w. **O** Wound appearance: 100% red, healthy granulation tissue with minimal drainage

x. Of the above statements, which would be considered "functional"? d, a, i, j, m, n, q, s, t, v, l

y. Of the above, which integrate or relate treatment, impairments, and function?

f, b, j, q,

2. Look at the initial examination and evaluation note that follows. Answer the following questions.

a. Which documentation format is being used: narrative, POMR, SOAP, or FOR?

b. Identify 3 pieces of subjective information.

c. Identify 3 pieces of objective data.

d. Based on the subjective and objective data, identify the activity limitations and participation restrictions.

e. Identify the PT diagnosis.

f. How did the PT describe the need for skilled care?

g. How did the PT demonstrate medical necessity?

h. In the next session, what information or data would the PT collect and record in an interim note to show changes in status or progress from the initial session? In what section(s) would the PT describe these changes?

i. What would be the most appropriate format for an interim note? Why?

j. What other individuals might be interested in looking at this patient's note(s)?

Date: March 1, 2012; 11.00

Pr: 27 y.o. male s/p (L) wrist & ankle fx; referred to outpatient PT to begin gentle wrist and ankle AROM and PROM and to begin gait training with crutches and (L) UE platform. PWB 50% (L) LE.

S: HPI: 4 wks. s/p fall (~ 25') from a logging truck landing on his (L) side (2/1/12). Pt. sustained fx of the (L) distal radius and ulna and (L) distal tibia & fibula. Pt. underwent ORIF for the wrist and ankle immediately after the injury. He was placed in a short-arm cast for the UE and short-leg cast for the LE. He was NWB on the (L) LE and has been unable to use crutches because he was not allowed to bear weight on the affected UE. At the time of the fall, the pt. also sustained a mild concussion. He was hospitalized for 5 days following the injury. While hospitalized he received inpatient PT to learn how to negotiate his w/c and transfer in/out bed. Both casts were removed yesterday and his ankle was placed in a removable splint. Reports taking ibuprofen PRN for pain.

C/C: Pain (pain scale = 2/10) & stiffness in (L) UE & LE with decreased functional use of both. Doesn't like using w/c for mobility. Unable to work. Requiring assist with self-care activities and home management.

L/S: RHD; lives with wife and 2 small children in single-level home with 2 steps at entrance and handrail on the (R). Prior to injury pt. was employed as a construction worker. He has been off work since the injury. Pt. is unable to drive and is relying on his wife and mother for transportation. No significant PMH or hx of fx. Reports being a nonsmoker and nondrinker. Family history is positive for OA.

Pt's goals: Return to previous level of function and RTW ASAP. Learn to ambulate with crutches

O: Systems review: Cognition and communicative ability are not impaired

AROM: (R) UE and LE are WNL; (L) shoulder, elbow, and hip are WNL; (L) hand: Pt. can perform a full fist but it is difficult because of edema; (L) Thumb IP, MCP, and CMC joints are WNL.

Wrist ROM			
	(L) wrist AROM (degrees)	(L) wrist PROM (degrees)	(R) wrist AROM (degrees)
Flexion	20	25	90
Extension	10	15	75
UD	10	15	35
RD	10	15	25
Supination	30	35	85
Pronation	40	45	75

Knee ROM			
	(L) knee AROM (degrees)	(L) knee PROM (degrees)	(R) knee AROM (degrees)
	0-100	0-110	15-0-145

Ankle ROM			
	(L) ankle AROM (degrees)	(L) ankle PROM (degrees)	(R) ankle AROM (degrees)
DF	−10 (from neutral)	0	20
PF	20	25	50
Inversion	5	5	50
Eversion	0	5	10

Strength: (R) UE & LE 5/5; (L) shoulder and hip 4/5; (L) elbow, wrist, knee, & ankle deferred because of acuity

Girth: Wrist figure 8 (R): 46 cm (L): 47.2 cm; ankle figure 8 (R): 52 cm (L): 54.1 cm

Sensation: (L) wrist and ankle intact to light touch and (=) when compared to the right

Circulation: 2+ at radial & dorsal pedal arteries on the (L)

Special Tests: N/A at this time due to acuity

Gait: Unable to ambulate at this time

Transfers: (I) Bed to/from chair, chair to/from toilet, sit to/from stand all NWB on (L) LE

Bed Mobility: (I) All areas.

Today's intervention and home instruction: AAROM for (L) wrist: flexion, extension, pronation, & supination to increase mobility; (L) ankle: DF and PF (also instructed in using opposite foot for self PROM) to increase mobility needed for gait; performed AROM for all digits and thumb to improve grip and decrease edema; instructed pt. in using ice, elevation, and compression wrapping for ankle and wrist; instructed pt. in use of crutches with platform for (L) UE, PWB 50% on (L) LE using step to gait pattern. Pt. required CGA × 1 for balance with crutches and gait pattern and verbal cueing. Pt. performed all ex. (I) & verbalized understanding of all precautions. Total treatment time 45 min following exam.

A: 27 y.o. RHD male 4 wks s/p fall sustaining (L) wrist and ankle fractures. PT dx: Impaired mobility in (L) UE and LE, edema, weakness, and newly healed fractures all limiting his ability to ambulate, drive, work, and manage his family and home tasks.

Problem list: Decreased AROM, PROM, strength, unable to ambulate, unable to perform (I) self-care or home management tasks, and unable to work at this time.

Rehab potential: Pt. demonstrates good potential for full recovery. No comorbidities that could affect outcome identified at this time.

Anticipated Goals and Expected Outcomes:

At the end of 2 weeks, the pt. will:

1. Increase AROM 10-15 degrees for the wrist, forearm, and ankle to allow improved mobility and self-care
2. Decrease edema by .5 cm for the wrist and ankle to allow improved mobility
3. Ambulate for unlimited distances with (L) UE platform PWB (L) LE (I)
4. Perform all self-care (I)
5. Perform a full fist without limitations to allow full grip during ADL and self-care

At the end of 16 weeks (d/c), the pt. will:

1. Have normal AROM of the wrist, forearm, & ankle (90-100% of opposite)
2. Grip & pinch strength will be 80-100% of (R)
3. Be (I) with all self-care and home management tasks
4. Ambulate (I) on all surfaces without an assistive device
5. Ascend/descend stairs (I) without an assistive device
6. Drive without restrictions
7. RTW at previous level of employment

P: Skilled services necessary to instruct pt. in safe and appropriate therapeutic exercise, use of assistive device, and gait pattern; also needed to safely progress gait and UE activity as ordered. Also will require instruction in strengthening exercises and retraining in functional mobility to prepare for return to normal lifestyle and RTW. See pt. 3×/wk for next 3 to 4 months for therapeutic exercise to improve mobility and strength for the hip, knee, shoulder, and elbow; gait training to increase (I) functional mobility to allow return to normal activities and participation. Will progress pt. as tolerated & according to physician orders. Pt. is in agreement with the above stated plan.

John Smith, PT

resides on a server or when a patient's health information will be transmitted electronically. HIPAA[31] provides federally regulated standards for handling individually identifiable health information during electronic transmission. This legislation requires that facilities adopt privacy policies and procedures for maintaining secure patient records so they are not accessible to unauthorized personnel.[32] HIPAA is discussed in more detail in Chapter 3.

REFERENCES

1. Quinn L, Gordon J. *Functional Outcomes: Documentation for Rehabilitation*. 2nd ed. Maryland Heights, MO: Saunders Elsevier; 2010.
2. Weed LL. *Medical Records, Medical Education, and Patient Care: The Problem-Oriented Medical Record as a Basic Tool*. Chicago, IL: Year Book Medical Publishers; 1970.
3. Dinsdale SM, Mossman PL, Gullickson G, Anderson TP. The problem-oriented medical record in rehabilitation. *Arch Phys Med Rehabil*. 1970;51:488-492.
4. Milhous RL. The problem-oriented medical record in rehabilitation management and training. *Arch Phys Med Rehabil*. 1972;53:182-185.
5. Feinstein AR. The problems of the "problem-oriented medical record." *Ann Intern Med*. 1973;78:751-762.
6. Mcintyre N. The problem-oriented medical record. *Br Med J*. 1973;2:598-600.
7. Reinstein L. Problem-oriented medical record: experience in 238 rehabilitation institutions. *Arch Phys Med Rehabil*. 1977;58:398-401.
8. Grabois M. The problem-oriented medical record: modification and simplification for rehabilitation medicine. *South Med J*. 1977;70:1383-1385.
9. Reinstein L, Staas WE, Marquette CH. A rehabilitation evaluation system which complements the problem-oriented medical record. *Arch Phys Med Rehabil*. 1975;56:396-399.
10. White JA. Managing care. Documentation: making it meaningful. *Phys Ther Case Rep*. 2000;3(2):78-79.
11. Clifton DW. "Tolerated treatment well" may no longer be tolerated. *PT Magazine*. 1995;3(10):24.
12. Abeln SH. Improving functional reporting (utilization review). *PT Magazine*. 1996;4(3):26, 28-30.
13. American Physical Therapy Association. *Guide to Physical Therapist Practice*. 2nd ed. Alexandria, VA: APTA; 2003.
14. American Physical Therapy Association. Defensible documentation. http://www.apta.org/Documentation/Defensible Documentation/. Accessed May 16, 2012.
15. Centers for Medicare & Medicaid Services. MDS 3.0 for nursing homes and swing bed providers. http://cms.gov/Medicare/Quality-Initiatives-Patient-Assessment-Instruments/NursingHomeQualityInits/NHQIMDS30.html. Accessed June 30, 2012.
16. Centers for Medicare & Medicaid Services. Inpatient rehabilitation facility PPS. https://www.cms.gov/Medicare/Medicare-Fee-for-Service-Payment/InpatientRehabFacPPS/index.html?redirect=/InpatientRehabFacPPS/. Accessed June 30, 2012.
17. Centers for Medicare & Medicaid Services. Home health PPS. https://www.cms.gov/Medicare/Medicare-Fee-for-Service-Payment/HomeHealthPPS/index.html. Accessed June 30, 2012.
18. Individuals with Disabilities in Education Act of 2004, PL 108-446. 108th Congress (2004). http://idea.ed.gov/download/statute.html. Accessed July 7, 2012.
19. Goldberg D. Sample IEP form: US Department of Education Model Form. http://www.specialeducationadvisor.com/iep-form/. Accessed June 30, 2012 .
20. Lewis DK. Do the write thing: document everything. *PT Magazine*. 2002;10(7):30-34.
21. Eng J. Tapping technology: computerizing clinical documentation. *PT in Motion*. Available at: http://www.apta.org/PTinMotion/2006/6/Feature/TappingTechnology/. Accessed June 30, 2012.
22. Vreeman DJ, Taggard SL, Rhine MD, Worrell TW. Evidence for electronic health record systems in physical therapy. *Phys Ther*. 2006;86:434-449.
23. Practice Fusion. What is HITECH. http://www.practicefusion.com/pages/HITECH.html/. Accessed July 1, 2012.
24. Centers for Medicare & Medicaid Services. Medicare & Medicaid EHR incentive program. https://www.cms.gov/Regulations-and-Guidance/Legislation/EHRIncentivePrograms/downloads/MU_Stage1_ReqOverview.pdf. Accessed July 7, 2012.
25. Centers for Medicare & Medicaid Services. EHR incentive programs. https://www.cms.gov/Regulations-and-Guidance/Legislation/EHRIncentivePrograms/index.html?redirect=/EHRIncentivePrograms/. Accessed July 1, 2012.
26. Garets D, Davis M. Electronic medical records vs. electronic health records: yes, there is a difference. http://www.himssanalytics.org/docs/WP_EMR_EHR.pdf. Accessed July 1, 2012.
27. MedicalRecords.com. The national digital records mandate: ARRA. http://www.medicalrecords.com/physicians/the-national-digital-medical-records-mandate-arra. Accessed June 30, 2012.
28. Shamus E, Stern D. *Effective Documentation for Physical Therapy Professionals*. 2nd ed. New York, NY: McGraw-Hill Companies Inc; 2011.
29. American Physical Therapy Association. APTA CONNECT: point of care for the physical therapist. http://www.apta.org/CONNECT/. Accessed July 7, 2012.
30. Abeln SH. Liability awareness. Reporting risk check-up. *PT Magazine*. 1997;5(10):38-42.
31. US Department of Health and Human Services. Health information privacy. http://hhs.gov/ocr/privacy/. Accessed January 28, 2012.
32. Ravitz KS. The HIPAA privacy final modified rule. *PT Magazine*. November 2002.

Chapter 6

Rules for Writing in Medical Records

Mia L. Erickson, PT, EdD, CHT, ATC

CHAPTER OUTLINE

Rules for Writing

CHAPTER OBJECTIVES

Upon completion of this chapter, the reader will be able to:

1. Describe the purpose of the APTA's *Guidelines for Physical Therapy Documentation of Patient/Client Management*.
2. Apply basic rules for documenting in medical records.
3. Describe what is meant by "unsubstantiated" terms written in a note.
4. Describe the importance of using skilled, medical language in medical records.
5. List ways to make notes more readable by others.
6. Correctly document late entries and addendums.
7. Correct errors written in a medical record.

KEY TERMS

addendum
authenticate
late entry

Erickson ML, Utzman RR, McKnight R. *Physical Therapy Documentation:*
From Examination to Outcome, Second Edition (pp 65-74).
© 2014 SLACK Incorporated.

As you start to look at the specific rules for writing in a medical record, remember the other important documentation points that have been described thus far. Look at the following bulleted list, as these points are necessary for documentation.

- The initial documentation includes patient impairments, activity limitations, and participation restrictions.

- The initial documentation describes how the impairments are contributing to the activity limitations and participation restrictions.

- The initial documentation describes the need and plans for skilled care and provides justification for why treatment is medically necessary.

- Interim notes describe how the intervention is bringing about change in impairment and function.

- All documentation details the therapist(s) skill(s) used during the examination or intervention.

- Documentation serves many purposes but the content must do the following:
  - Communicate
  - Demonstrate clinical problem solving
  - Support reimbursement and what was billed and needed for skilled services
  - Provide proof that care is or continues to be reasonable and necessary
  - Provide proof that care was skilled
  - Serve as a legal record

- Documentation is a record of patient/client management and it includes the examination, evaluation, diagnosis, prognosis, and interventions.

- PTs document patient/client management primarily through the initial documentation, interim notes (treatment notes and progress reports), and discharge summaries.

- Documentation also includes referrals, phone or electronic conversations, and communication with others.

In addition to these concepts required for documentation set forth in this text, the APTA provides the *Guidelines for Physical Therapy Documentation of Patient/Client Management* (Appendix A)[1] and Defensible Documentation.[2] These documents offer additional documentation guidance for physical therapy professionals across a variety of practice settings. The APTA documents are not intended to reflect documentation requirements in all practice areas, but they can serve as a "foundation" for developing documentation policies and procedures across a variety of unique and specialized settings.[1] Other authors have also reported specific rules for documenting in medical records.[3-11]

RULES FOR WRITING

Secure. Keep paper medical records and patient information in a secure, fireproof, locked file. Password-protect and securely store electronic records to prevent unauthorized access. Use laptops, tablets, or computers in a manner where they are not viewable by others or use privacy screen filters. Set computers to "time-out" after a period of nonuse.[12]

Authenticated. Date and authenticate (sign) all notations made in a patient's medical record. The PT authenticates the initial examination, evaluation, diagnosis, prognosis, and intervention plan. The PT and/or the PTA (where permissible by law) authenticate the treatment notes and the PT authenticates the progress reports and discharge summaries. The state's physical therapy practice act dictates how a signature appears in a written medical record. For physical therapy documentation, the PT and PTA generally provide their signatures, designation or credentials, and license number. Electronic signatures are also acceptable.

Complete. Place all relevant information related to the patient in his or her medical record. Include the patient's name, parent or guardian information (for minors), address, date of birth, health insurance information, emergency contact information, and physician information. Include all documentation reflecting the episode of care, such as consent forms, intake forms (eg, prior medical history, functional questionnaires), initial documentation, interim treatment notes, progress reports following regular reassessments, reevaluations when performed, discharge summaries, physician referrals, letters, communication notes, referrals to other health care providers, and any other pertinent information. Include attachments such as digital images or video. In a hospital setting, where all providers document in one medical record, one will find documentation completed by physicians, nurses, and other providers, as well as things such as lab reports and imaging studies.

Document special circumstances or situations in the patient's medical record such as cancellations, missed appointments, and verbal orders. Document reasons for *canceled or missed appointments or treatment sessions* whether initiated by the patient, the PT, the PTA, or another health care provider.

Example 6-1. Outpatient Cancellation Note

In an outpatient clinic, a snowstorm in December caused your patient to miss his 2 appointments. Document:

12/19/12: Patient canceled appointment because of weather. Rescheduled for 12/21. Sue Brooks, PT

12/21/12: Patient canceled appointment because of weather. Rescheduled for 12/23. Sue Brooks, PT

Example 6-2. Inpatient Cancellation Note

On a skilled nursing unit the nurse asks that you not work with a patient because the physician suspects the patient has a blood clot and is awaiting a Doppler study. Document:

12/12/11: Attempted to see Mrs. Smith this morning; however, nursing asked that we hold therapy because of possible blood clot, awaiting Doppler study. Will resume when cleared. Sue Brooks, PT

Document all *telephone or electronic conversations, such as email*, related to patient care. This could include conversations with the patent, the patient's family, the physician, other health care providers, or case managers.

Example 6-3. Telephone Call 1

You are working with a 24-year-old who was injured in a workplace accident. The patient's case manager for worker's compensation contacts you to determine the patient's status and progress. Document:

12/22/12: Spoke with patient's case manager today and provided update on strength, range of motion, and functional status as of reassessment performed on 12/20/12. Sue Brooks, PT

Example 6-4. Telephone Call 2

You are working with a patient with Alzheimer's disease who has recently undergone a right tibial open reduction and internal fixation because of a fracture. The orthopedic physician ordered "gait training non-weight bearing (R) lower extremity." However, because of the patient's confusion and inability to follow commands, she is unable to maintain these weight-bearing restrictions. You call the physician. Document:

12/01/12: Called Dr. Jones to make him aware that Mrs. Smith is unable to maintain weight-bearing restrictions because of confusion and inability to follow commands. Left message with nurse. Hold gait training until speaking with physician. Sue Brooks, PT

There may be times when the physician (or physician assistant) provides an order over the phone or in person. Document verbal orders in the following manner.

Example 6-5. Verbal Order

1/14/12: Verbal order received from Dr. Haines 1/14/12 @ 1:30 pm: Initiate whirlpool to patient's (L) foot. Sue Brooks, PT

The physician giving the verbal order then signs the order as soon as possible. Note, however, that PTAs do not take verbal orders or interpret referrals to physical therapy.

Document *unusual or unexpected situations or outcomes*. Some of these situations may also need an incident report. Completion of incident reports is discussed in another chapter. But, when an unusual event occurs, document the event, the patient's response in objective and measurable terms, your actions or response, and the outcome.

Example 6-6. Unexpected Situation

You are working with a 22-year-old woman who underwent a ligament repair to her right knee. She is performing resisted knee flexion strengthening and felt a "pop" in her knee. She immediately reported an increase in pain from 0/10 to 5/10. Document:

12/12/06: Pt. was performing right knee flexion exercises per standard protocol and felt a "pop" in her knee. Pain increased from 0/10 to 5/10. The patient was asked to discontinue her exercises for the day. Patient received ice to knee for 20 min. Called physician and left message with nurse for him to call back. After ice, patient reported a decrease in pain to 0/10 and she was able to ambulate without a limp. Will speak with physician about whether he wants to see the patient or continue per protocol. Sue Brooks, PT

Timely. Finish documentation in a *timely* manner, preferably as soon after the session as possible. First, the treatment session is fresh in your head and you are more likely to remember details sooner, rather than later. In addition, timely, completed documentation is necessary so that another therapist can treat your patient in the event of your absence. There are also administrative reasons for timely documentation. These include filing reimbursement claims and sending progress updates to others involved in the patient's care, including physicians, case managers, or insurance companies. Clinics and hospitals are likely to have policies in place requiring completion of all patient documentation within a given time frame.

Relevant, accurate, and logical. Ensure that entries in the medical record are relevant to the current condition or episode of care and reflect all necessary components of the session. Be as accurate as possible when documenting subjective or objective data. If subjective information comes from anyone except the patient, make sure you accurately document the person providing the information.

Example 6-7. Recording Subjective Information

The patient stated he wants to go to an inpatient rehabilitation facility prior to going home alone.

The child's parent indicated the need for a wheelchair assessment.

The child's teacher indicated the brace is causing a red spot on the right ankle.

After completing your documentation, review it to ensure it provides a precise, detailed depiction of the patient and situation as it occurred. Any clinician should be able to pick up one of the patient records and have a clear idea of what happened during the session.

Recall from Chapter 2 that documentation reflects the clinical problem-solving process used to arrive at the interventions. Provide a logical justification for the interventions being provided. For example, identify the relevant impairments, activity limitations, and participation restrictions in the subjective and objective data and highlight those in the problem list. Write a goal for each of the problems listed and aim the interventions at a specific goal.

Objective. Use *objective* language including *facts and observations.* Avoid making remarks about patients that cannot be substantiated by objective data. Remarks about a patient's response to a treatment should be given in objective, measurable terms (eg, "Patient's AROM increased from 80 to 110 degrees following treatment allowing the patient to sit more comfortably in a chair."). Avoid assessments about the patient's personality or their psychological status (eg, "Patient depressed."). Although you may be trying to provide additional information about the patient, you must be very careful not to make a judgment for which you are not qualified.[9] Also, avoid subjective terms such as "appears" and "seems to be."[13] Finally, use professional, neutral language and do not write unnecessary remarks about the patient, family member, caregiver, or another provider. You should not look as though you are taking sides on any issues between the patient and another individual (eg, a physician or case manager).

Clear and concise. Entries must be clear and concise, but also be thorough and provide sufficient documentation to accurately reflect the encounter, demonstrate that services were skilled, and prove that the intervention is reasonable and necessary. Never leave out pertinent information or a rationale for services for the sake of brevity. As you are learning to write medical records, err on the side of being too lengthy or verbose. You can learn to "skim down" later after you get more experience and better understand necessary information.

Consistent. In general, use similar types of documentation throughout the patient's episode of care at your facility—that is, forms, templates, formats, flow sheets. Use a similar format or template for documenting all body parts or diagnoses. Also, use similar formats or templates for writing interim notes, progress reports, reevaluations, and discharge summaries so that reviewers and other health care providers can easily locate necessary information. It also helps another PT or PTA find information quickly. This is important for a provider who is treating a patient for the first time.

Legible. Handwriting that is not legible has potential to lead to medical errors. In addition, third-party payers have been known to deny claims based solely on the fact that they could not read the provider's handwriting. If this is a problem, consider dictating your notes and using a transcription service or converting to an electronic record.

Scientific. In most cases, use professional *scientific, medical terminology.* Avoid "nonskilled language" such as "the

patient walked . . .." Instead, use descriptive, functional, and/or medical language, such as "provided gait and transfer training . . .." There may be times, however, when more lay language is appropriate. This might be during a pediatric, school-based session where a copy of the documentation is provided to the parents or guardians at the end of the day.

Skilled. Describe the unique skills or assist you used or provided to facilitate the patient during the session(s) that go above and beyond what could be provided by an untrained individual.[14] Describe the assist, cues, and specific technique(s) used. This can be difficult to do, especially when trying to be concise. Use your knowledge of the intervention to describe what you are doing during the session. A description of *how* your unique and sophisticated skills are used provides insight to the patient's need for skilled services and is a requirement for documentation. Look at the following examples.

Example 6-8. Skilled Language 1

DO NOT WRITE:

"Patient performed therapeutic exercise for 15 min."

INSTEAD:

Describe why the patient performed the exercises.

"Patient performed strengthening exercises for the left quadriceps and hamstrings for 15 min to improve knee control during gait. Tactile cues were required for quadriceps facilitation."

Example 6-9. Skilled Language 2

DO NOT WRITE:

"Patient ambulated 15 min requiring moderate assist of 1."

INSTEAD:

"Patient ambulated 15 min requiring moderate assist of 1 to facilitate (R) quadriceps during the swing phase of gait to increase knee extension and step length."

Also, in the initial documentation, include any plans and reason for skilled treatment that will be done.

Medically necessary. In the initial documentation and progress notes, justify why the physical therapy is medically necessary. In addition, describe why the patient needs a particular intervention. Proving medical necessity can be difficult but it is necessary. Document any medical diagnosis or condition (including physical therapy diagnosis) that prevents the patient from performing the intervention independently. Use your scientific knowledge of the intervention and describe *why* you are needed to provide a particular treatment. You may also include known evidence as a justification for a particular treatment. Include the

		AROM (degrees)	PROM (degrees)
(R) Shoulder	Flexion	140	155
	Extension	10	15
	IR	50	55
	ER	45	55
(R) Elbow	Flexion	140	140
	Extension	225	220
	Supination	80	n/a
	Pronation	80	n/a

Table 6-1

Example of Active and Passive Range of Motion Documented in a Table

justification for every new treatment you initiate throughout the episode of care.

Example 6-10. Medically Necessary Interventions

Patient will receive passive stretching to increase joint range of motion necessary for overhead activity.

Patient will receive gait and balance training to increase endurance and safety needed for independent household ambulation.

Patient will be educated on the proper use of the orthoses to protect healing tissues and prevent skin breakdown.

Patient will receive manual traction to remove pressure from nerve root and decrease pain.

Patient requires passive range of motion performed by a therapist because of new rotator cuff repair. The patient is unable to perform the treatment himself because of contralateral extremity range-of-motion limitations.

Patient-centered. Document using *third person* because the emphasis is on what the patient can do or does. Look at the following example.

Example 6-11. Third-Person Language

DO NOT WRITE:

I ambulated the pt. 50 min and provided minimal assistance ×1 for balance and verbal cueing for upright posture because of postural sway.

INSTEAD:

The patient ambulated 50 min requiring minimal assistance ×1 for balance and verbal cueing for upright posture because of postural sway.

There are times, however, when using the first person is unavoidable. This usually occurs after special situations and you are describing what happened in the narrative format.

Organized. *Use headings* to group relevant information together, to indicate new sections, and to designate important patient information. Headings make the note easier to read and identify necessary information. Examples of appropriate section headings and subheadings can be found in Table 5-1. In instances where there is a great deal of data that can easily become confusing to the reader, it is appropriate to *use tables, columns, or lists.* Tables are valuable when documenting range of motion or strength on several joints (Table 6-1).

Formatted. Finally, document according to widely accepted rules for writing in medical records. Write with *black or blue permanent ballpoint ink.* Erasable ink or pencil should never be used. Be aware of your spelling, language, and grammar. In addition, use only *industry-standard, facility-approved, medical terminology, symbols, and abbreviations* (see Appendix D). Do not overuse abbreviations because they can be misinterpreted and confusing, especially if a reader is unfamiliar with the abbreviations. When reading others' notes, realize some abbreviations have more than one meaning (eg, PT = physical therapist and prothrombin time). Read the entire note to determine the context of the abbreviation, so that you can interpret it appropriately. Check with your facility regarding acceptable abbreviations and their use.

Avoid skipping lines in the record. Begin your note, starting with the date of service, on the line immediately below the prior entry. Do not skip lines in the middle of your notes. Skipping lines could allow someone to come back at a later date and fraudulently add in information.

If you must come back to a record later and document something that you may inadvertently omitted, then document the information as a *late entry or addendum.* Never rewrite or inappropriately add information to the original note. A chart entry is considered a "late entry" when other health care providers have documented after your original documentation or when enough time has elapsed so that the date you are writing the late entry is different from the original documentation. In this case, the late entry should be placed in chronological order for the date that *it is written* and be identified as a "late entry." An explanation for the late entry should also be provided.[3] Sign the late entry as you would any other documentation.

If you immediately realize you have forgotten to write something that should have been included, write an addendum. An addendum is written immediately following the original documentation. Identify the additional information with the heading, "Addendum:" following the original documentation without skipping a line. Sign the addendum as you would your original documentation.

If you make an error, correct it by placing a single straight line through the text. An individual reading the note should still be able to read the original text. Provide your initials and date next to the error. Never use correction fluid or erasable ink in a medical record.

Example 6-12. Errors

The patient ~~ambulated~~ (MLE 2/18/12) transferred with minimal assist × 1 for stabilizing the left knee to prevent buckling.

When documentation of patient care requires *more than one page*, make sure subsequent or additional pages include the patient's name, patient or chart number, and the date. Transition the information like the following example.

Example 6-13. Multiple Pages

"Continued next page-Sue Brooks, PT." Then, on the next page, write: "Continued from previous."

Rules for writing more specific aspects of the documentation are provided in subsequent chapters.

REVIEW QUESTIONS

1. What components of patient care should be reflected in physical therapy documentation?

   Everything - if it's not documented it didn't happen

2. What is the purpose of the APTA's *Guidelines for Physical Therapy Documentation of Patient/Client Management* and Defensible Documentation?

3. Give one example (other than those given in the chapter) of how documentation from examination to discharge can be *consistent*.

   Be consistent in the benchmark tests given to the patient to judge improvement

4. Give one example (other than those given in the chapter) of a statement that would be "unsubstantiated" or an unqualified judgment of a patient.

   Give specific ROM numbers instead of saying "the patient's ROM improved"

5. What ink colors are most appropriate for writing in medical records?

   black or blue

6. What is the purpose of using medical language and terms describing your unique contribution to assisting the patient? *to show that the pt. requires skilled care by a PT that can't be done by a different healthcare provider*

7. How much time should elapse between treating the patient and documenting the encounter?

8. What does the term *authenticate* mean?

Sign

9. What factors differentiate a "late entry" from an "addendum?"

"late entry" - document written after the treatment date
"addendum" - forgetting something you needed to include

10. Examine your state's physical therapy practice act.

a. Are there regulations or requirements for documenting physical therapy services? If so, what are they?
b. Are there regulations or requirements for PTs that are different for PTAs regarding documentation? If so, what are they?
c. Are PTAs required to have notes cosigned by a PT? How does this vary, or differ, depending on practice setting?
d. How do documentation regulations or requirements in your state's practice act differ from the Model Practice Act issued by the Federation of State Boards of Physical Therapy (www.fsbpt.org)?

APPLICATION EXERCISES

1. For the following entries, indicate those that are <u>inappropriate</u> by writing an "I" next to the item. Describe why they are inappropriate. Also, indicate the items that would be considered "skilled." Of those that are unskilled, how could they be improved?

a. _I_ The patient ~~walked~~ 50'. *ambulated*
b. _I_ This patient requires skilled services. *for what?*
c. _I_ Patient stated that she enjoys coming to physical therapy.
d. __ Patient complains of pain in the (L) knee following exercise after last visit.
e. __ <u>AROM:</u> (R) shoulder flexion 160 degrees; abduction 120 degrees. *need range*
f. __ Patient performed quad sets, glut sets, and straight leg raises. *how many?*
g. __ Patient walked around the physical therapy gym twice. *specifics*
h. _ Patient reported compliance with his home exercise program and reports increased range of motion.
i. __ Patient is demonstrating excessive hip abduction with his prosthesis during ambulation.
j. __ <u>Gait:</u> 100' with hemi-walker with minimal assist ×1 for trunk support and minimal assist ×1 for advancing the (L) lower extremity.
k. __ <u>Transfers:</u> Bed to/from chair with minimal assist of 1 to support the trunk because of poor balance.
l. __ <u>Ther Ex:</u> Performed 20 repetitions all exercises.
m. __ <u>Bed mobility:</u> Rolls supine to and from side lying with minimal assist of 1 for support of lower extremity fracture.
n. __ HEP: Instructed the patient in a home exercise program to be performed daily.
o. __ The patient reported to physical therapy today in a wheelchair with his leg on an elevated leg rest, which is the same way he had been transported to physical therapy all week.

2. Write the following information in a clear, concise manner, as it would appear in the medical record. Use the SOAP format and include headings where appropriate.

a. The patient walked 75 feet in the hallway of the hospital one time with the therapist lightly touching her back for balance because of dizziness. She used a front-wheeled walker.
b. The patient's strength was 3/5 for the right biceps and 4/5 for the right triceps.
c. Upon arrival to therapy, the patient told you that she has been doing her HEP without any problems and really feels like her ability to reach into an overhead cupboard has improved.
d. The patient said that her pain was 3/10 on a pain scale.
e. The patient demonstrated the following range of motion measurements: active range of motion for the right elbow was 130 degrees flexion and 10 degrees of hyperextension.
f. Knee active range of motion was 100 degrees flexion and lacking 10 degrees of extension.
g. The patient propelled his wheelchair around the hospital (250 feet), outside on the sidewalk, and up and down 3 ramps with you providing verbal reminders on trunk positioning for going up and down the ramp.

h. The patient walked 50 feet using the wide-based quad cane and the ankle-foot orthosis (AFO) on the right ankle. She needed minimal assistance of 1 to swing the right leg to prevent getting her toes caught on the floor. The patient was able to put her AFO on and remove it independently. She required verbal cues to check her skin for any irritated areas after she removed it.

i. During a busy morning in a hospital, you were working with a patient who told you that she was going to be discharged and wanted home health services, primarily physical therapy. After writing the note and completing your morning treatment sessions, you realize that you did not document your patient's desire for home physical therapy. What should you do? How would you document this entry into the chart? Where should this information be placed?

j. After documenting a patient's passive range of motion of the right shoulder, you realize that you made an error. It should have been 125 degrees, not 152 degrees. Demonstrate how to correct this mistake if you find it immediately.

3. Identifying Documentation Errors

Read the following notes and list problems that you identify.

Example #1—Initial Documentation

Therapist: John Smith, PT

Physician: Dr. Harris

Date: November 7, 2012

Diagnosis: s/p (R) rotator cuff repair and acromioplasty

ICD-9: 840.4

Functional Impairments: Patient is limited in any activity requiring overhead or active movement of the (R) UE.

Date of Onset: Patient fell and injured (R) shoulder on October 2, 2012. Surgery was November 1, 2012.

Next MD Appointment: November 14, 2012

Diagnostic Tests: MRI. See attached report.

History/Relevant Subjective: Patient fell on October 2, 2012, landing on the (R) UE. After fall, he complained of significant pain and sought medical attention. MRI revealed partial thickness tear of rotator cuff. Underwent repair to (R) rotator cuff by Dr. Harris on November 1, 2012. Patient reports point tenderness along the spine of the scapula that is limiting him from performing his ADL. Patient has not been sleeping well and reports pain at 8/10 on the pain scale. Patient has difficulty raising his arm overhead because of pain; however, pain decreases when arm is placed on his stomach. Patient would like to improve independence in ADL without pain and perform home management tasks.

Objective: Asymmetrical arm movement during gait. AROM: flexion 30 degrees, abduction 90 degrees, IR 80 degrees, ER 15 degrees. PROM: flexion 60 degrees, abduction 100 degrees, IR 70 degrees, ER 20 degrees. Resistive testing found flexion, abduction, and ER weak and painful. Electrodes placed over the (R) shoulder for premodulated electrical stimulation 80 to 150 Hz × 20 minutes with ice.

Assessment: s/p (R) rotator cuff repair and acromioplasty

STGs:

1. Decrease pain from 6/10 to 4/10 within 2 to 3 weeks

2. Increase PROM 10 to 20 degrees in flexion, abduction, and ER

Discharge Goals:

1. Independently perform ADL within 6 to 8 weeks

2. Decrease complaints of pain to 0/10 within 6 to 8 weeks

3. Obtain functional ROM within 6 to 8 weeks

Rehab Potential: Good

Interventions To Be Used: Modalities, ultrasound, electric stimulation, laser. Manual therapy, PROM, stretching, and joint mobilizations. Therapeutic exercises and activities will be performed per protocol.

Frequency and Duration of Treatment: Two to three times per week for 8 to 12 weeks at discretion of physician to increase strength of glenohumeral and scapular muscles, ROM, and decrease pain.

— — —

Example #2—Initial Documentation

Date: March 1, 2012

Subjective/History: Pt. c/o mild, achy pain in the upper and lower thoracic region. Pain is noted with sitting, especially with a slumped posture. Pt. is RHD. Pt. is involved with youth basketball.

Objective: Standing Posture: Right thoracic convexity and left lumbar convexity. Displays kypholordotic curvature. Right rib hump. PSIS and iliac crests are equal heights bil. Right foot more pronated than left. AROM with flexion: pt. veers to the right with full ROM. Displays full extension with a hinge point at L4-L5. Bil. side flexion and rotation are full. Pt. hamstrings are minimally tight. Quadriceps are not tight. Both hip abductors and adductors are 3/5. Paraspinals are 3/5 with difficulty. Pt. rx today consists of initial evaluation and therapeutic exercise of shoulder ER, horizontal abduction, and D2 flexion/extension pattern with yellow exercise band. Pt. performed 1 set of 10 reps. HEP consists of 10 × 3 sets 2 to 3 times per day of each exercise. Pt. educated on proper posture and the use of a lumbar roll for correct posture. Pt.'s mother present for treatment session.

Assessment: 14 y.o. girl with scoliosis. Referred by CRNP after X-rays. Postural dysfunction and weakness.

STGs: Within 1 to 2 weeks, the pt. will

1. Be independent with a HEP
2. Improve strength to 4/5 on convex side
3. Improve flexibility on concave side

Discharge goals: Within 3 to 4 weeks, the pt. will

1. Be independent with a home exercise, maintenance, and prevention programs
2. Have a good understanding of the importance of correct, erect posture, and maintaining exercise following therapy
3. Be independent with lumbar stabilization techniques and understand the importance of neutral pelvis

Plan: See pt. in clinic 2 times per week for 4 weeks. For therapeutic exercise, postural education, lumbar stabilization training, neuromuscular reeducation, manual therapy, and pt. education.

Suzy Smith, PT

— — —

Example #3—Initial Documentation

Date: March 1, 2012

History: 15 y.o. girl with (B) Achilles tendon pain starting last August. PMH: (B) patellofemoral pain syndrome. Referred by physician last week for physical therapy 3 times per week for 1 month with dx of (B) equines. No meds. C/C: Increased pain in (B) Achilles with repetitive jumping and after sports. Home situation: Lives with her parents and attends school. Pt.'s goal is to return to jumping pain free and be ready for softball season. Pain level 3/10 right and 4/10 left.

O:	AROM:	Right	Left
	DF	2 degrees	6 degrees
	PF	WNL	WNL
	Inv	WNL	WNL
	Ev	WNL	WNL
Strength:	DF	5/5	5/5
	PF	5/5	5/5
	Inv	5/5	5/5
	Ev	5/5	5/5
Girth:	1-1/2' from calcaneus	32-1/2 cm	33-1/4 cm
Edema:		(–)	(–)
Tenderness:		(–)	(–)
Sensation:		Intact to light touch	Intact to light touch

Today's Tx: Education-condition and what we will be doing in therapy to help correct it. Ther Exercise: Gastroc-soleus stretching 3 × 30 s each; supination and pronation in standing to fatigue; towel curls

PT Diagnosis: Practice Pattern 4F: Impaired joint mobility, motor function, muscle performance, and range of motion associated with localized inflammation

A: 15 y.o. girl c/o (B) Achilles pain after activity such as jumping and recreational activities

Problem list:

1. Unable to run
2. Unable to jump
3. Unable to participate in recreational activities
4. Pain level 3/10 right; 4/10 left

STGs: In 2 weeks, pt. will

1. Have decreased pain after activity to 2/10
2. Be able to tolerate fast-paced walking × 20 min
3. Increase DF to 8 degrees right and 10 degrees left

Discharge goals: In 4 weeks, the pt. will

1. Be free of pain in (B) Achilles
2. Return to normal recreational activities without c/o pain
3. Have ROM WNL
4. Be independent and compliant with HEP

Plan: See pt. 3 times per week for 2 weeks for

1. Functional training
2. Flexibility
3. HEP

Joe Thompson, PT

— — —

Example #4—Initial Documentation

Physical Therapy Report

Date: 4/5/12

S: A 67 y.o. man brought to ER 4/2/05 with unrelenting chest pain and tightness. Admitting dx: MI. Now 1 day s/p CABG ×3. No current complaints. Lives in 2-story home with wife; bedroom on second floor with 1 flight of steps and a handrail on the right. Retired but enjoys active lifestyle, including farming. Pt.'s goal to return to previous active lifestyle.

O: From the chart: Height: 6'2"; Weight: 345#. BP, 135/75; HR, 78 bpm; RR 10. Transferred out of bed to chair with moderate assist × 2. Ambulation not assessed at this time secondary to protocol. Performed 10 reps CABG postop exercise.

A: 1 day s/p CABG ×3. Problem: limited mobility STGs: In 2 days, pt. will ambulate in the hallway with supervision and transfer in/out of bed with minimal assist. Discharge goals: In 5 to 7 days, pt. will ambulate

150' to 200' with supervision and transfer independently.

P: See pt. bid for CABG protocol.

John Smith, PT

REFERENCES

1. American Physical Therapy Association. Guidelines: Physical Therapy Documentation of Patient/Client Management BOD G03-05-16-41. http://www.apta.org/uploadedFiles/APTAorg/About_Us/Policies/BOD/Practice/DocumentationPatientClientMgmt.pdf. Accessed May 16, 2012.
2. American Physical Therapy Association. Defensible documentation. Available at: http://www.apta.org/Documentation/DefensibleDocumentation/. Accessed May 16, 2012.
3. Abeln SH. Liability awareness. Reporting risk check-up. *PT Magazine*. 1997;5(10):38-42.
4. Arriaga R. Liability awareness. Stories from the front: documentation and clinical decision making: a real-life scenario illustrates some basic risk-management principles. *PT Magazine*. 2002;10(5):46-49.
5. Goode N. The reliable resource: physical therapy documentation. *PT Magazine*. 1999;7(9):30-31.
6. Inaba M, Jones SL. Medical documentation for third-party payers. *Phys Ther*. 1977;57:791-794.
7. Redgate N, Foto M. Pay by the rules: avoid Medicare audits and reduce payment denials with a sound strategy and proper documentation. *Phys Ther Prod*. 2003;October/November:28-30.
8. Scholey ME. Documentation: a means of professional development in physiotherapy. *Physiotherapy*. 1985;71:276-278.
9. Schunk CR. Liability awareness. Advice for the new physical therapist: here are some keys to avoiding risk once you've made the transition from student to practitioner. *PT Magazine*. 2001;9(11):24-26.
10. White JA. Managing care. Documentation: making it meaningful. *Phys Ther Case Rep*. 2000;3(2):78-79.
11. Lewis DK. Do the write thing: document everything. *PT Magazine*. 2002;10(7):30-34.
12. Erickson ML, McKnight R. *Documentation Basics: A Guide for the PTA*. 2nd ed. Thorofare, NJ: SLACK Incorporated; 2012.
13. Clifton DW. "Tolerated treatment well" may no longer be tolerated. *PT Magazine*. 1995;3(10):24.
14. Hester H. Preparing for medical review: auditing your documentation. Presented at: Combined Sections Meeting of the American Physical Therapy Association; February 2012; Chicago; IL.

Chapter 7

Documenting Patient Histories and Interviews

Ralph R. Utzman, PT, MPH, PhD

CHAPTER OUTLINE

CHAPTER OBJECTIVES

Upon completion of this chapter, the reader will be able to:
1. List sources of information for historical data.
2. Differentiate between the Problem and Subjective sections of the note.
3. Identify types of data that should be recorded in the Problem and Subjective sections of a SOAP note.

Erickson ML, Utzman RR, McKnight R. *Physical Therapy Documentation:
From Examination to Outcome, Second Edition* (pp 75-82).
© 2014 SLACK Incorporated.

4. Discuss how historical data inform the clinical decision-making process.

5. When given information collected from a patient history, organize the information in logically sequenced Problem and Subjective sections.

6. Describe how the Problem and Subjective sections of the note will vary between initial notes, interim/progress notes, and discharge summaries.

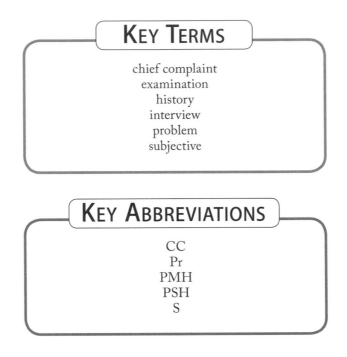

KEY TERMS

chief complaint
examination
history
interview
problem
subjective

KEY ABBREVIATIONS

CC
Pr
PMH
PSH
S

According to the Patient/Client Management Model in the *Guide to Physical Therapist Practice*,[1] the first step in physical therapy care is examination. A patient examination begins with a thorough patient history. During history taking, the therapist gathers information from the patient; family; other providers; and the medical record about the patient and his or her health condition, impairments, activities, and participation. This step is vital in identifying the patient's need for physical therapy services.[2,3] The history provides information that helps the therapist choose the appropriate tests and measures to perform. The patient's goals, expectations, and educational needs are also identified. This chapter reviews the contents and structure for documenting the patient history.

ORGANIZING THE INFORMATION

In the SOAP note format, historical information is divided into 2 distinct sections (refer to Figure 7-1). The first, called Problem (often abbreviated Pr:), contains information found in the medical record, physician referral, reports or results of laboratory tests, etc. The Problem section may be quite long if there is extensive information already available in the medical record. This is frequently the case in hospitals or other institutional settings. The second section is called Subjective (usually abbreviated S:) and contains information given by the patient, family, or caregiver.

"Subjective" refers to information that is gathered from a secondary source rather than from a direct measurement or observation. Subjective information is gathered during the patient interview and provides insight into what the patient knows about his or her condition and its impact on functional activities and participation.

In each major section of the note, subheadings are often used. These subheadings allow for organization of the information presented so that specific data can be located more easily by the reader. The *Guide for Physical Therapist Practice*[1] describes several categories of historical data, which are summarized in Table 7-1. Any or all of these might appear in the Problem or Subjective section of the note depending on the source of information.

The subheadings used in each examination note will vary based on the patient's situation and the setting in which care is delivered. Some general guidelines of information to include in each subheading follow.

General Demographics

The initial note should include basic information about the patient's age, gender, and ethnicity. If the patient's primary language is not English, it should be noted here as well. If the patient has been referred to physical therapy by another provider, it is customary to include this information with the statement of the referral (see "Writing Problem and Subjective" section on p. 79).

Table 7-1

Categories of Historical Data Recorded in a Physical Therapy Examination

Subheading	*Type of Information*
General demographics	• Age, language, gender, ethnicity
Functional status and activity level	• Current and prior functional status, including ADL and IADL
Occupation and employment	• Current and prior community and work/school activities
History of current condition	• Chief complaints—concerns that led patient to seek physical therapy • Current treatment by other providers • Mechanism of injury • Date of onset • Onset and pattern of symptoms • Patient and family/caregiver goals and expectations • Patient and family/caregiver perceptions and emotional response to current clinical situation
Medications	• All medications the patient is taking, both for this problem and others • Include prescription and over-the-counter medications and supplements
Other tests and measures	• Laboratory tests • Radiology tests
Past history of this condition	• Prior interventions and their outcomes
Past medical/surgical history	• Prior hospitalizations and surgeries • Preexisting medical and health conditions (comorbidities)
Growth and development	• Developmental history • Hand/foot dominance
Family history	• Familial health risks
Living environment	• Devices and equipment • Home layout • Community characteristics • Projected discharge destination
Social history	• Cultural beliefs and behaviors • Family/caregiver resources • Social interactions and support systems
Health status	• General perception of current health • Physical, psychological, role, and societal function
Social habits	• Behavioral health risks • Level of physical fitness

Data compiled from Figure 2 in *Guide to Physical Therapist Practice*. (From American Physical Therapy Association. *Guide to Physical Therapist Practice*. 2nd ed. Alexandria, VA: APTA; 2003:36.)

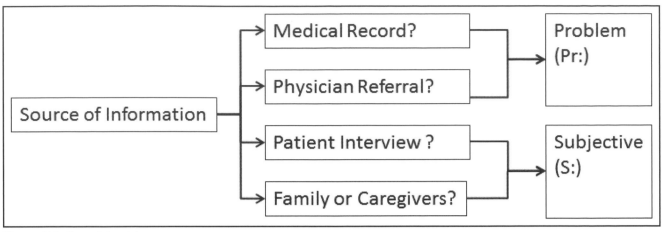

Figure 7-1. Organizing history.

History of Current Condition

The patient should be asked about his or her chief complaint. The chief complaint (C.C.) is the reason the patient is seeking physical therapy or health care services. The patient may express the chief complaint as a symptom, such as pain, dizziness, etc. Patients will also often state the chief complaint in terms of activity limitations (eg, pain with lifting) or participation restrictions (eg, unable to work). The date of onset, mechanism of injury, and behavior of symptoms (location, duration, severity, how symptoms change with activity) will provide important clues about the patient's problem and further guide the examination process. It is important to note what treatment has been provided for the patient so far and whether these treatments have helped. This portion of the patient interview should lead to a discussion of the patient's goals and expectations for physical therapy and set a foundation for the patient-therapist relationship.

Functional Status and Activity Level

You should carefully note the person's level of activity and participation, both currently and before the injury/illness that brought him or her to physical therapy. This is important information to establish the need for physical therapy and to guide the remainder of the examination. Documenting good information about functional status will help determine which tests and measures should be performed later in the examination. In many cases, the expected outcome of therapy is to return the patient to his or her previous level of function, so documenting this information will be helpful in establishing a prognosis later in the note.

Clinical Tests and Measures

It is important for the PT to document clinical tests and measures that have been performed, such as clinical laboratory and radiology reports. Whenever possible, this information should be gathered from or confirmed by the medical record and documented in the physical therapy note. These reports give vital information about

the patient's diagnosis, clinical medical condition, and precautions that may need to be followed. For instance, a patient with low hemoglobin and hematocrit levels may not tolerate physical activity, so the therapist may need to delay interventions until these levels return to normal.

Even though clinical test results may be available elsewhere in the patient's medical record, it is still important for the therapist to document them in his or her documentation. Test results contribute to the therapist's overall evaluation of the patient and often impact the physical therapy plan of care. Also, documenting this information in the physical therapy note will allow the PTA or others who are participating in or reviewing the physical therapy care of the patient to have ready access to the information. If the test result report is lengthy, it is acceptable for the therapist to summarize the key findings in the physical therapy note and refer readers to the full report.

Example 7-1. Documenting Results of Medical Tests

Clinical Tests: Chest x-ray 11/14/2012 10:25 am indicates atelectasis in the right lower lobe. Refer to radiology notes for further details.

Past Medical/Surgical History (PMH/PSH)

Many of our patients come to us with multiple medical conditions. These comorbidities may impact the patient's progress in therapy. Consider, for example, 2 patients who undergo knee replacement surgery. One patient has a history of asthma and requires a slightly longer course of therapy to build respiratory endurance after the surgery. The other patient has a history of diabetes and requires close monitoring of blood glucose levels during exercise. Each of these patients' plans of care will need to take the comorbidities into account when considering intervention duration, parameters, and precautions. Whenever possible, this information should be gathered from or confirmed by the medical record. In settings where this is not possible, this information must be gathered through careful, thorough patient interview.

Medications

You should note every medication the patient is taking, including those for other health conditions. Besides helping alleviate patient's symptoms or treat other health conditions, some medications may cause side effects or alter the patient's response to exercise or other activities. Be sure to include any over-the-counter medications and supplements.

Occupation and Employment

Documentation should include information on the patient's current occupation. Even if the patient is not formally employed, the requirements of the patient's social roles (student, mother, homemaker, retiree) should be documented. Documentation of the patient's work, school, home, and leisure activities provides important insight into the patient's prior level of function and contributes to setting goals for therapy.

Growth and Development

PTs provide care for patients across the life span and patients' activities and participation change with their life stages. Some patients access physical therapy to address developmental disabilities. In these cases, it is important to accurately document a thorough developmental history with special emphasis on participation and function in life tasks. This will help guide selection of appropriate tests and measures for the objective portion of the exam.

Documentation of hand dominance is also important, especially in the case of upper extremity impairment. Treatment strategies and patient expectations may be different based on whether the injured extremity is dominant or nondominant.

Family History

Family health risks should be identified and documented as a mechanism for screening and prevention. Patients with a family history of heart disease, diabetes, stroke, or high blood pressure, for example, may need referral to a physician for further screening and intervention. For example, a 64-year-old woman is referred to physical therapy for evaluation of dizziness and balance problems. During the patient interview, the therapist notes the patient's mother and grandfather both developed type 2 diabetes later in life. The patient reports that her dizziness is not affected by body position or head movement, and the therapist confirms this in her examination. The therapist refers the patient to her physician for further workup, who determines the patient does have diabetes.

Living Environment and Social History

In inpatient settings, PTs play a key role in discharge planning. We assess the patient's activity limitations and participation restrictions and make clinical judgments to predict the patient's functional status at discharge. As the patient prepares to go home, it is important to note the layout of the patient's home, adaptive equipment the patient has available, and support available to the patient from the community. For patients in the outpatient setting, this information is also important to guide the treatment plan and optimize the patient's function in the home and community.

Physical therapists are expected to provide care that is culturally appropriate for the patient.[1] Along with the living environment, it is important to note the patient's health-related cultural beliefs, social interactions, and available support system.

Health Status and Social Habits

Another piece of important functional information is the patient's perception of his or her health. The goal of physical therapy is to maximize the patient's movement-related activity and optimize participation in his or her social roles. Patients' perceptions of their health can be impacted by physical, emotional, psychological, and social determinants. Discussing the patient's perception of his or her current and expected level of health can further discussions of the patient's goals for physical therapy.

Many health-related social habits can affect function and quality of life. It is important to note the patient's level of fitness, dietary habits, and use of substances such as tobacco and alcohol. A patient who engaged in regular physical activity before an illness or injury may tolerate a more aggressive exercise protocol than a patient who was previously sedentary. Patients who have poor dietary habits or who smoke may experience slower healing that may, in turn, impact the rate of recovery. Identifying these lifestyle habits can help guide goal setting, identify opportunities to improve physical fitness, and clarify needs for referrals for smoking cessation or dietary consultations.

WRITING PROBLEM AND SUBJECTIVE

The initial examination note should start with the time and date. It is customary to write the time using a 24-hour clock ("military time"); you may use a regular 12-hour clock as long as you clearly indicate am or pm. If the note is handwritten in a record that includes multiple practitioners, a title is needed so that readers know what discipline the note is representing (ie, "Physical Therapy") and what type of note they are reading (eg, "Initial Evaluation Note"). Next, start with the first major heading, which is "Problem" (or Pr:). This heading should appear on the very next line below the date, time, and title. *Never* leave blank lines in handwritten notes.

At a minimum, the Problem section should include basic demographics of the patient, medical diagnosis, and referral information. This can be done in 1 or 2 narrative phrases. For example:

Example 7-2A. Stating the Problem

11/2/2012 PHYSICAL THERAPY INITIAL EVALUATION
PROBLEM

67 y.o. woman s/p right THA referred 11/1/2012 for "Evaluate and Treat, partial weight-bearing right lower extremity" by Dr. David Jones.

Note that the passage includes the date of referral, the name of the physician, and a direct quote of the referral. If the patient has multiple diagnoses and/or a complex referral, you could separate the parts of this passage with subheadings, then follow with other information from the chart review. For example:

Example 7-2B. Stating the Problem

11/2/2012 PHYSICAL THERAPY INITIAL EVALUATION
PROBLEM

67 y.o. woman

Medical Diagnosis: right THA, right lower lobe pneumonia.

Referral: 11/1/2012 for "Evaluate and Treat, partial weight-bearing right lower extremity" by Dr. David Jones.

Clinical Tests: Chest X-ray 11/14/2012 10:25 am indicates atelectasis in the right lower lobe. Refer to radiology notes for further details.

Next, the note should document information provided by the patient and/or the patient's family or caregivers. This begins with the new heading of "Subjective," or "S:" As with the Problem section, information can be organized using subheadings as appropriate. Here is an example of the Problem and Subjective sections of an evaluation note for a patient in an acute care hospital.

Example 7-3. Problem and Subjective

11/2/2012 10:45 PHYSICAL THERAPY EVALUATION NOTE
PROBLEM

24 y.o. man referred by Dr. Jones 11/1/2012 0730 for "ROM exercises and gait training WBAT (L)LE. Patient must wear Bledsoe brace while walking."

Diagnosis: ACL repair (L) knee yesterday.

Meds: Percocet prn. Last taken 2 hours ago.

SUBJECTIVE

HPI: Pt injured (L) knee 2 weeks ago while playing intramural flag football. Pt. was moving to avoid an opponent when he was struck on the LLE by another player. He was seen in the emergency room and referred to orthopedics.

PMH: No previous surgeries.

CC: Pt reports pain (L) knee. The pain increases with movement.

Living Environment/Social: The patient lives in an upstairs apartment. He has 10 steps leading up to the apartment, with a handrail on the right going up. He has a roommate who can help with cooking and cleaning, but the patient will need to be independent in ADL.

Occupation: Pt. is a third-year PT student.

Functional Status: Prior to injury, pt. was active in intramural sports. Since the injury, pt. has been using axillary crutches.

Pt. Goals: The patient wishes to return to recreational sports. The patient is scheduled to go on clinical internships next semester, and will need to be independently mobile without assistive devices by mid-February.

Recall that the key difference between the Problem and Subjective sections is the source of the information. In the above example, if the patient had told the therapist about what medications he was taking, the information would have appeared under Subjective instead of Problem.

If the patient is self-referred (ie, the patient has accessed physical therapy without a physician referral) and you are relying solely on patient report, then you should omit the Problem section entirely. The following is an example of documentation of a history taken from a patient who was not referred by a physician.

Example 7-4. Documentation of Subjective Information from a Self-Referred Patient/Client

11/2/2012 14:30 PHYSICAL THERAPY EVALUATION NOTE
SUBJECTIVE

Chief Complaint: 55 y.o. woman presents with complaints of vertigo.

HPI: Patient experienced episode of severe vertigo 1 week ago when turning over in bed. The vertigo lasted for less than a minute and was accompanied by nausea and vomiting. She now reports feeling "off balance" and dizzy.

Symptoms are worse when she looks up, when she turns her head quickly, or when she bends over.

PMH: No previous surgeries. Patient reports history of hypertension, treated by Dr. Jennifer Jackson.

Medications: Captopril

HPI: Patient experienced episode of severe vertigo 1 week ago when turning over in bed. The vertigo lasted for less than a minute and was accompanied by nausea and vomiting. She now reports feeling "off balance" and dizzy. Symptoms are worse when she looks up, when she turns her head quickly, or when she bends over.

PMH: No previous surgeries. Patient reports history of hypertension, treated by Dr. Jennifer Jackson.

Medications: Captopril

Living Environment/Social: The patient lives in a 2-story home with her husband and daughter. There are 10 steps between levels with a handrail on the right side.

Occupation: Patient is an accountant and plays golf weekly.

Functional Status: Prior to onset, patient was independent in all mobility and ADL. Since onset, she has been afraid to drive and is unable to golf. She notices that she holds onto walls and door frames when walking, and feels unsteady when climbing stairs.

Pt. Goals: The patient wants to alleviate her symptoms, improve walking, and resume driving.

DIFFERENT TYPES OF NOTES

The length and contents of Problem and Subjective sections will differ based on what type of note is being written. In an initial evaluation, you will be reporting extensive historical information. Therefore, the Problem and Subjective sections may be quite long and will include many of the subheadings listed above. In subsequent notes, the Problem and Subjective sections are typically much shorter.

Interim Notes and Progress Reports

After the initial evaluation note, information in the Problem section need not be repeated in subsequent notes. However, new test reports or other medical record information may become available. This can occur if the patient's medical status has changed, if medications have been added or deleted, or if new medical or radiologic tests are completed. In these cases, it is appropriate to include a brief Problem section prior to the Subjective section of the interim note.

The patient interview process is not isolated to the patient's first visit. On return visits, the therapist must record the patient's response to the previous treatment. Such entries may involve response of pain or other symptoms, and should include changes (either positive or negative) in functional status. Including the patient's perceptions regarding progress helps establish the medical necessity of the care being provided. The therapist should also ask questions about the patient's adherence to home exercise programs and record the information here. Again, things the patient says are documented under the Subjective section. As in initial evaluation notes, subheadings may be used to organize information. If the section is brief, however, subheadings can be omitted.

Example 7-5. Subjective Report in a Progress Note

11/3/2012 09:15 PHYSICAL THERAPY PROGRESS NOTE

S: Pt reports mild pain (L) knee. Pt. used ice during the night to help with pain and swelling.

Pt. performed quads sets and straight leg raises this morning, and has been getting up to the bathroom with crutches and family assist.

The Discharge Summary

The Hx: section may include a brief summary of the patient's history and progression of care. The S: section will contain information similar to that contained in the progress note. The patient should also be asked to reflect on his or her total progress since care was initiated. Comparing the patient's statements regarding function at discharge to that at the time of initial examination can help determine whether goals related to impairments, activities, and

REVIEW QUESTIONS

1. Describe the types of historical information that should be documented in the medical record.

demographics, medications, history of current condition, past medical history, family/social history, living environ.

2. What are the sources of information in the Problem (Pr:) and Subjective (S:) sections of a note?

Pr: medical record, physician referral S: patient interview, family/caregiver

3. Discuss the relationship between historical data and the tests and measures portion of the examination.

4. Outline an appropriate structure for the Problem and Subjective sections of a note documenting an initial patient encounter/evaluation.

5. Outline an appropriate structure for the Problem and Subjective sections of a note documenting an interim/daily treatment session.

6. Outline an appropriate structure for the Problem and Subjective sections of a note documenting a discharge summary.

participation are met. They may also aid in justifying any follow-up care planned after discharge.

Application Exercises

1. Provide the subheading for each of the following types of subjective data.
   a. Symptoms, such as pain *history of CC*
   b. Age *general demographics*
   living environment c. Number of steps to get into the patient's home
   surgical history d. Type of surgery performed
   e. Patient's ability to get in/out of bed *Functional Status*
   f. Ability to ambulate before surgery *history CC*
   g. Work tasks *occupation + employment*
   past history h. Reports of seeking care from a chiropractor
   i. Patient's prior health status *past med. history*
   j. Hand dominance *growth + development*
   k. Patient's mother died of a stroke *fam. history*
   l. Results of blood work *other tests / measures*

2. For each of the examples in exercise 1, how would you determine whether the information should be documented in the Problem or Subjective section of the note? Which source do you think would be the best for each item?

3. Write each of the following in a clear, concise manner.
   a. The patient told you that her pain was a 6 on a 0 to 10 scale.
   b. The patient told you she feels dizzy when shopping; dizziness is worst walking down the aisle of a supermarket.
   c. The patient's husband told you that his wife has fallen at home several times. They had to call an ambulance to get her up off the floor.
   d. The patient told you that she gets tired and short of breath when vacuuming, cleaning the bathroom, and doing other household tasks.

e. The patient told you that she lives alone. She has neighbors and friends from church who stop by. Her daughter, who lives in another state, calls her 2 to 3 times per week.

4. Review the Problem and Subjective sections of the following note written about a patient seen in an outpatient clinic. Is any critical information missing? Does the note include information about activity limitations and participation restrictions? What questions would the physical therapist ask to gain missing information? What is the best source for this information?

11/30/2012 14:30 PHYSICAL THERAPY EVALUATION NOTE
PROBLEM
24 y.o. man referred by Dr. Tracy Frum for "Evaluate and treat"
Diagnosis: low back pain
SUBJECTIVE
CC: Pt. reports pain in the right lower back and buttock.
HPI: Patient injured at work 2 weeks ago while lifting boxes.
PMH: Tonsillectomy in 1994.
Living Environment/Social: The patient lives in an apartment with 2 roommates.
Occupation: Patient is a graduate student. He has a part-time job with UPS.
Pt. Goals: Reduce back pain.

References

1. American Physical Therapy Association. What are physical therapists, and what do they do? In: *Guide to Physical Therapist Practice.* 2nd ed. Alexandria, VA: American Physical Therapy Association; 2003:31–42.
2. Quinn L, Gordon J. *Functional Outcomes Documentation for Rehabilitation.* St. Louis, MO: Saunders; 2003.
3. Stewart DL, Abeln SH. *Documenting Functional Outcomes in Physical Therapy.* St. Louis, MO: Mosby-Year Book; 1993.

Chapter 8

Documenting Objective Information

Ralph R. Utzman, PT, MPH, PhD and Mia L. Erickson, PT, EdD, CHT, ATC

CHAPTER OUTLINE

CHAPTER OBJECTIVES

Upon completion of this chapter, the reader will be able to:

1. Identify types of data that should be recorded in the Objective section of the SOAP note.

2. Discuss the purpose of the Review of Systems.

3. Discuss how objective data are used to inform the clinical decision-making process.

4. Differentiate between measurements of impairments of body structure/function and measurements of functional activity limitations.

5. Discuss characteristics of tests and measures: general versus specific, self-report versus performance-based.

6. When provided data collected during a patient examination, arrange the data into a logically sequenced Objective section.

Erickson ML, Utzman RR, McKnight R. *Physical Therapy Documentation:*
From Examination to Outcome, Second Edition (pp 83–88).
© 2014 SLACK Incorporated.

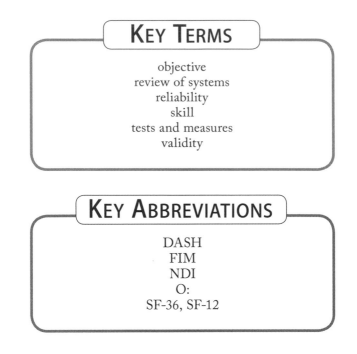

The previous chapter described documentation of a patient's history information gathered from review of the medical record, physician referral, and patient interview. Next, the PT performs a physical examination of the patient and may initiate intervention. The Objective (or O:) section of the note contains data derived from the physical examination and a description of the intervention performed during the current treatment session.

OBJECTIVE CONTENTS

Whereas the Subjective section of the note contains information relayed by the patient or caregivers, the Objective section provides facts that can be observed or measured. These facts are generally presented without judgments or evaluation—analysis of the data occurs in a later section of the note. The Objective section includes results of a brief screening examination called the Review of Systems, followed by detailed Tests and Measures. If interventions are provided, they should be presented as well. As with the Problem and Subjective sections, use of subheadings can help to emphasize important information and to make specific facts easier for readers to find.

Review of Systems   Systems Review

The Review of Systems is defined by the *Guide to Physical Therapist Practice*[1] as a "brief or limited examination" that includes screening various body systems for anatomical or physiological impairments. The purpose of the Review of Systems is to establish, along with data from the chart review and patient interview, the need for the physical therapy examination and to guide the PT's selection of more specific tests and measures.[1]

The Review of Systems should be brief but, at a minimum, it should include screenings of the cardiovascular, integumentary, musculoskeletal, and neuromuscular systems along with the patient's cognitive status, communication abilities, and affect. If the PT finds no impairments in a particular system, the therapist simply notes "unimpaired" under the appropriate subheading. If evidence of impairment is found, the findings are briefly noted and the reader is referred to the Tests and Measures section for further details. An example of the Review of Systems follows.

Systems Review

Example 8-1. Review of Systems

Systems Review

Cardiovascular/Pulmonary: Unimpaired. At rest, HR, 80; BP, 110/70; RR, 16

Integumentary: Unimpaired

Musculoskeletal: Gross strength and ROM (B)UE, (R)LE unimpaired. Impaired strength and ROM (L)LE.

Neuromuscular: Unimpaired

Communication/Cognition: Pt. alert & oriented ×4. Pt. wears hearing aid.

Tests and Measures

The Tests and Measures portion of the Objective section provides results of the physical examination of the patient. The PT selects tests and measures based on the information collected from the chart review, patient interview, and Review of Systems.[1] Thorough and accurate documentation of tests and measures provides baseline data about the patient's impairments, activity limitations, and participation restrictions. This baseline serves as the starting point for developing a patient prognosis and plan of care and demonstrating patient improvement over time. Selecting appropriate tests and measures involves deciding what aspects of "health" you wish to measure, then matching measurement tools appropriately. PTs should also have adequate background knowledge of the measurement properties associated with tests and measures, including reliability (test-retest and interrater), validity, responsiveness, and the test's ability to measure change. A listing of tests and measures used by PTs can be found in Chapter 2 of the *Guide to Physical Therapist Practice*.[1]

Measuring Impairment

Consider identifying impairments important to your patient population and determine appropriate tools to measure the impairments. If you are interested in examining range of shoulder motion in individuals with adhesive capsulitis, then goniometric measurements may be an appropriate outcome measure. On the other hand, consider a patient with lateral epicondylitis. These patients rarely have limited range of motion, so goniometric measurements may not be appropriate. It may be more appropriate to measure pain during gripping or lifting tasks. Other impairments often measured include strength, sensation, endurance, reflexes, and balance.

Measuring Function

Generic versus specific measures. Finch et al[2] described the use of both generic and specific tools for measuring function. Generic measures, or general health status questionnaires, are not specific to any one pathology or diagnosis. Generic measures, such as the Functional Independence Measure (FIM),[3] are used to assess "overall" aspects of the individual's functional capacity, such as walking, transferring, bathing, and dressing. Generic measures are appropriate for both healthy and unhealthy populations and allow clinicians to assess physical function alone, or physical function combined with societal integration.[2] Some generic measures are also used to evaluate emotional response(s) to injury and psychosocial issues through subscales. In addition to the FIM, other popular generic measurement tools include the Short-Form Health Survey (SF-36),[4] its shortened counterpart the SF-12,[5] and the Sickness Impact Profile.[6]

Specific measures of function include pathology (disease)-specific, body part (body region)-specific, and patient-specific measures. Pathology-specific measurement tools include items that are geared specifically to assess function and disability for individuals with a given pathology, such as the Arthritis Impact Measurement Scales[7] and the Fibromyalgia Impact Questionnaire.[8] In body part- or region-specific tools—such as the Disabilities of the Arm, Shoulder, and Hand (DASH) Questionnaire,[9] the Neck Disability Index (NDI),[10] and the Oswestry Low Back Pain Questionnaire[11]—patients are scored based on a set of predetermined tasks using the involved body part (eg, writing or turning a key on the DASH). Patient-specific measurement tools allow each patient to identify his or her own set of functional tasks he or she may be unable to perform because

of the injury or illness. In using a patient-specific measure, the patient is not provided with a predetermined list of functional tasks. For example, the Patient-Specific Functional Scale[13] requires the provider to ask the patient to identify 3 to 5 important activities that he or she is having difficulty with or is unable to perform because of the illness or injury. Then, the patient is asked to rate the level of difficulty on a scale of 0 to 10, with 0 indicating "unable to perform" and 10 being "able to perform at preinjury level."[13]

Authors have identified strengths and weaknesses of both generic and specific measurement tools. First, generic health measures allow comparisons to be made across different patient cohorts and have relatively "good measurement properties."[2(p17)] Nevertheless, generic measures may hide or mask functional problems specific to certain pathologies. Some patients seen in an outpatient orthopedic setting may score very high on generic health measures. For example, the patient with lateral epicondylitis could obtain a perfect score on the FIM yet be unable to work because of pain and pain-induced weakness. Generic or general health measurement tools may also be "less sensitive to change than more specific measures"[2(p17)] and may "hide sensitive clinical changes."[14(p1)] In these cases, the instrument does not capture relevant patient changes because of interventions.

Strengths of specific measurement tools have been identified. Specific tools measure functional problems often unique to a pathology or body part, and thus "capture" specific problems for that population. Questions are targeted at identifying disability due to a specific pathology, or injury to a body part, rather than evaluating general health-related quality of life. More specific functional tasks that appear on these types of questionnaires are generally not included in a generic tool. In addition, functional changes occurring as a result of an intervention may be seen more clearly using a specific tool rather than a generic quality-of-life questionnaire. Weaknesses of specific tools, however, has been described by Finch et al.[2] These authors reported that comparison of scores on specific tools is limited to patients with the same condition or problem of the same body part—that is, patients with rotator cuff syndrome or patients with acute low back pain. Finally, a specific measure may not capture general quality-of-life changes.[2]

Patient performance versus self-report. In performance-based outcomes measures, the patient is required to perform a set of functional tasks, such as the FIM. In using the FIM, the patient is assessed according to his or her ability to (1) perform self-care skills (eg, feeding and dressing), (2) control bowel/bladder function, (3) transfer, (4) move (eg, gait and stair climbing), (5) communicate, and (6) interact socially, including memory and problem solving.

Function and disability assessments can also rely on "self-report." In self-report measures, the patient completes a questionnaire, rating his or her overall performance on a predetermined set of functional tasks. An example of a patient self-reported functional measure is the Oswestry Low Back Pain Questionnaire, often used to assess the functional status of patients with back pain. Other examples of self-reported questionnaires include the SF-36, the NDI, and the Patient-Rated Wrist Evaluation.[12]

Describing Interventions

Physical therapy intervention involves 3 interrelated components: communication and coordination with other health care providers, patient-related instruction, and procedural interventions. Documentation should clearly describe how you have coordinated the patient's care with other members of the health care team. The importance of recording this documentation was covered previously in Chapter 3. Some examples are as follows:

narrative

Example 8-2. Documentation of Communication

- Called Dr. Smith to recommend radiograph of (R) ankle.
- Notified Becky Perry, RN, that the patient became nauseous during treatment; Ms. Perry came to Pt.'s bedside at the conclusion of the session.

Similarly, document any instructions that you may have given. This includes discussions of **informed consent** (see Chapter 3) in which you discuss the planned interventions with the patient. Do not forget to document instructions given to family members or other caregivers. Besides documenting what instructions were given, provide details on the teaching methods used and the patient's (or caregiver's) response to the instruction. Some examples are as follows:

Example 8-3. Documenting Instructions and Informed Consent

- Discussed purposes and procedures for selective wound debridement, as well as risk of bleeding or infection. Discussed use of sterile technique to reduce these risks. Discussed alternatives (whirlpool, wet-to-dry dressings) that will require more frequent therapy and carry similar risks. Pt. was given the opportunity to ask questions before giving consent to the procedure.
- Instructed patient in prone-on-elbows positioning 30 seconds × 5 reps, 3 times daily. Patient was able to demonstrate this exercise correctly without verbal cues.
- Taught the patient's husband techniques for guarding the patient during home balance exercises. After a demonstration of proper body position and hand placement, patient's husband was able to safely guard the patient.

Document all procedural interventions and describe all the parameters associated with the treatment. For example, when describing an exercise session, the therapist documents the type of equipment used, the joint(s) and movement(s) involved, the mode (active, passive, resisted), the level of resistance, the number of repetitions and sets, and length of rest periods between exercises. For patients with cardiovascular impairments or poor endurance, documentation of vital signs before, during, and after exercise is warranted. When documenting the use of physical and electrotherapeutic agents, include the type of modality and all of the parameters (waveform, duration, temperature, frequency, intensity, etc) of the modality.

When documenting interventions, the therapist should demonstrate the **skill** required to perform the treatment provided. In order to be reimbursed, the documentation must prove the treatment provided required decision-making capacity and the unique skills of a qualified provider. If such skill is not accurately described, the reader might assume that the patient could have completed the task or exercise without help, or that a family member or other health care worker could have provided the assistance with less cost.

Example 8-4. Skilled versus Unskilled Language

Unskilled language: "The patient ambulated with a walker for 20 feet, PWB LLE, with minimal assistance."

Skilled language: "The patient ambulated with a walker for 20 feet, PWB LLE. The patient required minimal assistance for walker placement, tactile cues to maintain PWB LLE, and instruction on proper gait sequence," shows that the therapist's intervention was skilled. The therapist was providing ongoing assessment, education, and cues for safety that require the skills and judgment of a PT.

Counting Minutes

Medicare, insurance companies, and other third-party payers are reviewing therapists' documentation and billing with increasing scrutiny. They often compare the bills submitted with care documentation to look for fraud and abuse. If a clear relationship cannot be made between the care documented and the services billed, the payer may deny the claim. In most care settings, PTs are required to document the number of actual minutes spent on each type of activity or treatment performed with each patient. This can be accomplished by noting the number of minutes spent on various activities in the Objective section.

DIFFERENT TYPES OF NOTES

Just like the Problem and Subjective sections of the note, the contents of the Objective section will vary based on the patient's health condition, functional abilities, and care

---

Example 8-5. Documenting Objective Information

O: <u>Systems Review:</u>

<u>Cardiovascular/Pulmonary:</u> Unimpaired. At rest, HR, 80; BP, 110/70; RR, 16.

<u>Integumentary:</u> Unimpaired

<u>Musculoskeletal:</u> Gross strength and ROM (B)UE, (R)LE unimpaired. Impaired strength and ROM (L)LE.

<u>Neuromuscular:</u> Unimpaired

<u>Communication/Cognition:</u> Pt. alert & oriented ×4. Pt. wears hearing aid.

<u>Functional Status:</u> Sit-stand with minimal assistance of 1 for initiation of forward trunk movement and hip extension. Ambulates 10 feet/30 seconds with walker, min A of 1 for advancement of walker and to maintain TDWB LLE. After ambulation, HR, 106; BP, 128/76; RR, 22.

<u>AROM:</u> (L) knee flexion 5-75°, hip flexion 0-95°.

<u>Strength:</u> (L) hip flexors and knee extensors 3+/5, (L) ankle plantarflexion and dorsiflexion 4+/5.

<u>Today's Treatment:</u> Gait and transfer training as described above for 15 minutes. Therapeutic exercise for a total of 20 minutes, including AROM (L) hip & knee flexion 10 reps, cued patient to hold movement at maximum hip/knee flexion for 5 seconds with each repetition. Instructed Pt. in supine (L) straight leg raises 3 sets of 10 repetitions. Pt. was instructed to perform these exercises in his room later this afternoon. Pt. was able to demonstrate each exercise correctly.

---

setting. The length and contents of the Objective section will vary based on the type of note (eg, initial evaluation, progress/interim note, discharge summary).

The initial note will include all of the results of the physical examination as well as a description of any interventions performed in the initial session. Depending on the patient's functional status and impairments, this section may be rather long and the use of subheadings is recommended.

Include any new measurements or examination results at each interim visit. Make sure descriptions of interventions show skill and progression of the treatment program. These notes might be shorter than the Initial Evaluation Note, so use of subheadings is optional.

Every patient should be reexamined on a regular basis and at the end of care. Documentation of these reexaminations should include updated information on the

Example 8-6. Use of Tables

Measurement	Initial (10/15/2005)	Today
(L) Knee AROM flexion	10 to 55 degrees	5 to 95 degrees
(L) Quadriceps strength	3–/5	4/5

REVIEW QUESTIONS

1. Define the types of information that should be included in the Objective section of a SOAP note.

    Systems review, functional status, range of motion, strength, today's treatment

2. List the types of data obtained during the systems review process. How is this information used for clinical decision making?

    vitals (BP, HR), integumentary system, neuromuscular, cognition

3. How are data from tests and measures used in decision making?

    Serves as a baseline for prognosis and plan of care

4. Compare and contrast impairments (of body structure and function) and function (activity limitation and participation restriction). Give examples of measurements for each.

5. Compare and contrast generic (general health), disease-specific, and patient-specific instruments. Give positive and negative aspects of each.

6. Compare and contrast patient performance and self-report questionnaires. Give positive and negative aspects of each.

patient's functional status and impairments. The format for documenting these results is the same as the initial examination. In addition, some clinicians find it helpful to list initial and current status side by side in table format, as follows:

APPLICATION EXERCISES

1. Outline the contents of the Objective section of an initial examination note. How might the contents be different in an interim/progress note and a discharge summary?

2. Review the list of tests and measures in the *Guide to Physical Therapist Practice*. Choose 1 category and identify 1 test/measure that can be used to collect data for that category. Does the test provide information regarding impairments or function? Is it a self-report measure or a performance measure? Research the reliability and validity of the test/measure you selected.

3. Write the following statements in a more clear and concise manner as it would appear in the medical record.

   a. The patient had trouble standing up from a seated position. The therapist applied tactile and verbal cues for the patient to lean forward and push up with her hands and provided minimal assist for balance on initial standing.

   b. The patient's active range of motion for right shoulder abduction was from 0 degrees to 80 degrees; the patient reported pain at end range.

   c. During the systems review, the measurements taken for blood pressure were 130/90, heart rate 98 bpm, oxygen saturation was 98%, and respiratory rate was 12 breaths/min.

4. While examining a patient who has been experiencing falls, the following information was collected. Using the outline you created in Application Exercise 1, organize the information into a concise Objective section.

Patient's blood pressure is 128/78 and her heart rate is 72 bpm. She has an abrasion on her forehead slightly to the left of midline. She walks with slow steps and a wide base of support, holding onto walls and doorways for support. The only gross active range of motion impairments you notice is a limitation in shoulder flexion bilaterally, and gross strength is symmetrical. The patient is alert and oriented and follows instructions accurately. She wears bifocal glasses. The following tests and measures were performed during the examination. The patient's gait speed is 0.6 m/s. She scores 16/24 on the Dynamic Gait Index. Static standing balance on firm surface with arms crossed and feet together, she can stand for 30 seconds without assistance; the same position with eyes closed elicits backward trunk sway after 12 seconds. On a foam surface with arms crossed and feet together, she exhibits posterior trunk sway after 18 seconds;

with her eyes closed standing on foam, she loses her balance after 5 seconds and needs assist to avoid a fall. She scores 42 out of 56 possible points on the Berg Balance Scale. Deep tendon reflexes are 2+ throughout. Sensation to light touch is normal using monofilament testing. No nystagmus is noted with movement or at rest. Active range of motion of right shoulder flexion is limited to 0 to 125 degrees, and the left to 0 to 115 degrees. Passive range of motion of right shoulder flexion is 0 to 130 degrees, left to 0 to 120 degrees with capsular end feel. Quadriceps strength and hip abductor strength are 4/5 bilaterally via manual muscle test.

REFERENCES

1. American Physical Therapy Association. What types of tests and measures do physical therapist use. In: *Guide to Physical Therapist Practice*. 2nd ed. Alexandria, VA: APTA; 2003.

2. Finch E, Brooks D, Stratford PW, Mayo NE. *Physical Rehabilitation Outcome Measures*. 2nd ed. Philadelphia, PA: Lippincott Williams & Wilkins; 2002.

3. Uniform Data System for Medical Rehabilitation. About the FIM system. http://udsmr.org/Default.aspx. Accessed January 10, 2013.

4. Ware JE Jr, Snow KK, Kosinski M, Gandek B. *SF-36 Health Survey Manual and Interpretation Guide*. Boston, MA: The Health Institute, New England Medical Center; 1993.

5. Ware JE Jr, Kosinski M, Keller SD. A 12-item short form health survey: Construction of scales and preliminary tests of reliability and validity. *Medical Care*. 1996;34:220-233.

6. Bergner M, Bobbitt RA, Carter WB, Gilson BS. The Sickness Impact Profile: Development and final revision of a health status measure. *Medical Care*. 1981;19:787-805.

7. American College of Rheumatology. Arthritis impact measurement scales (AIMS/AIMS2). http://www.rheumatology.org/practice/clinical/clinicianresearchers/outcomes-instrumentation/AIMS.asp. Accessed January 10, 2013.

8. American College of Rheumatology. Fibromyalgia Impact Questionnaire (FIQ). http://www.rheumatology.org/practice/clinical/clinicianresearchers/outcomes-instrumentation/FIQ.asp. Accessed January 10, 2013.

9. Institute for Work and Health. Disabilities of the arm, shoulder, and hand. http://www.dash.iwh.on.ca/system/files/dash_questionnaire_2010.pdf. Accessed December 30, 2012.

10. Vernon H, Mior S. Neck Disability Index: a study of reliability and validity. *J Manipulative Physiol Ther*. 1991;14:409-415.

11. Fairbank JCT, Pynsent PB. The Oswestry Disability Index. *Spine*. 2000;25:2940-2952.

12. MacDermid JC, Tottenham V. Responsiveness of the disability of the arm, shoulder and hand (DASH) and patient-related wrist/hand evaluation (PRWHE) in evaluating change after hand therapy. *J Hand Ther*. 2004;17:18-23.

13. Westaway MD, Stratford PW, Binkley JM. The patient-specific functional scale: validation of its use in persons with neck dysfunction. *J Orthop Sports Phys Ther*. 1998;27:331-338.

14. Hart DL. What should you expect from the study of clinical outcomes? *J Orthop Sports Phys Ther*. 1998;28:1-2.

Chapter 9

Writing the Assessment and the Plan

Mia L. Erickson, PT, EdD, CHT, ATC and Rebecca McKnight, PT, MS

CHAPTER OUTLINE

CHAPTER OBJECTIVES

Upon completion of this chapter, the reader will be able to:

1. Outline the information recorded in the Assessment and Plan sections of a SOAP note.

2. Describe the relationship between the evaluation and the examination.

Erickson ML, Utzman RR, McKnight R. *Physical Therapy Documentation:*
From Examination to Outcome, Second Edition (pp 89-103).
© 2014 SLACK Incorporated.

3. Differentiate between a medical diagnosis and a physical therapy diagnosis.

4. Integrate a physical therapy diagnosis into the documentation.

5. Discuss the use of "rehabilitation potential" in clinical documentation.

6. Integrate comorbidities, complications, and complexities into the clinical documentation.

7. Describe the clinical decision-making process used in establishing a patient prognosis.

8. Construct short- and long-term goals in the form of behavioral objectives that include all pertinent information.

9. Integrate scientific evidence on tests and measures into a goal.

10. Organize given information into a properly structured assessment and plan.

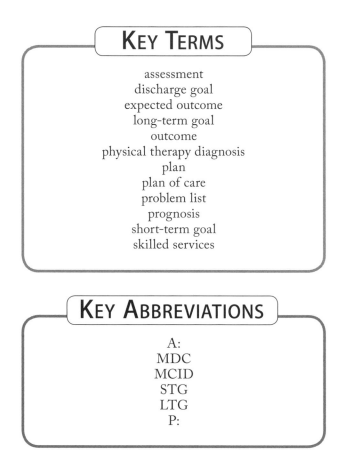

KEY TERMS

assessment
discharge goal
expected outcome
long-term goal
outcome
physical therapy diagnosis
plan
plan of care
problem list
prognosis
short-term goal
skilled services

KEY ABBREVIATIONS

A:
MDC
MCID
STG
LTG
P:

Following the examination, the PT reviews the data collected (history, systems review, and tests and measures) and synthesizes the information to determine the physical therapy diagnosis, prognosis, and plan of care. According to the *Guide to Physical Therapist Practice*,[1] this clinical reasoning process is known as the *evaluation*. At first glance, the examination and evaluation appear to be linear in nature—meaning, the examination points to the evaluation, which then leads to the diagnosis, prognosis, and plan of care (Figure 9-1). In reality, however, there is often interplay between the examination and the evaluation. It is also important to recognize the dynamic nature of these processes.[1]

Throughout the examination, the PT makes clinical judgments on various pieces of subjective and objective data. Depending on the data, the PT probes further, or moves on in a different direction. This is somewhat of a step forward-step back approach, allowing the PT to rule in and rule out various impairments, activity limitations, and participation restrictions. Jones[2] described this clinical reasoning process as "cyclic" and used the "hypothetico-deductive method" to describe the decision-making process used during a physical therapy examination. Using this strategy, one establishes a hypothesis and then uses questioning, tests, or measures to prove or disprove it. During the examination and evaluation processes, the PT develops an initial hypothesis of the clinical problem(s) and proceeds with the examination by choosing questions, tests, or measures that confirm or deny the working hypothesis. Each question or test will provide information that will feed back into the process until sufficient information is obtained to make a clinical decision about the patient and the intervention plan.[2] The PT documents these clinical judgments and decisions within the Assessment and Plan sections of the SOAP note.

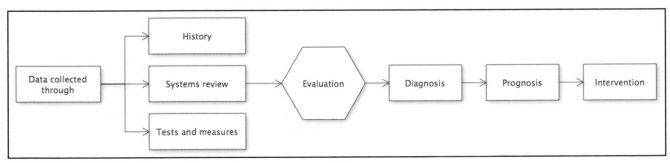

Figure 9-1. Linear view of clinical decision making in physical therapy.

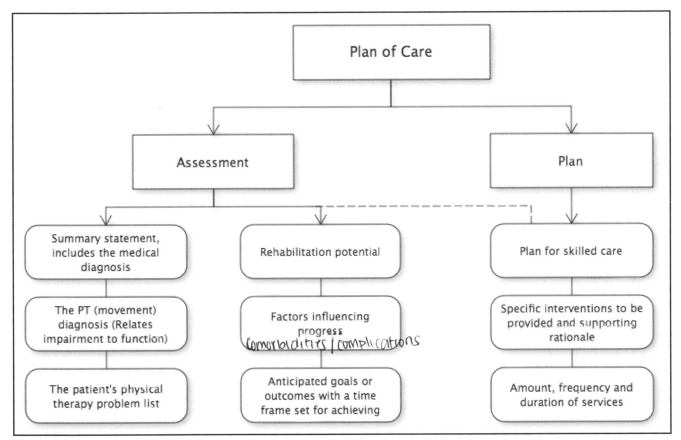

Figure 9-2. Template for the initial Assessment and Plan (Plan of Care).

DOCUMENTING THE ASSESSMENT AND PLAN (PLAN OF CARE)

Collectively, the Assessment and Plan (A: and P:) are often referred to as the plan of care, or treatment plan. Some third-party payers, or insurers, have specific guidelines for information included in a plan of care,[3] and it is the PT's responsibility to stay abreast of documentation guidelines and requirements for care plans since documentation requirements change frequently and vary across states, payers, and settings. A template for creating a plan of care can be found in Figure 9-2 and can be used when learning this aspect of documentation. This template provides components of A and P sections of the initial documentation; however, many variations exist and different facilities may have different policies for placement of information within the initial documentation. Once the components that are necessary have been learned, one can be flexible in the arrangement and placement within the documentation to comply with various facility, or even payer policies. In addition, the authors of the text chose to organize the contents using the SOAP structure but realize that in the clinical setting, these sections may be written as one document, called the plan of care (see p. 152 and Appendix C). As stated previously, the emphasis should be on the contents and quality of documentation.

The Assessment and Plan are often the most difficult sections of the note to write. It is the PT's chance to articulate and summarize the reason for the intervention plan, realizing that others (eg, PTAs, third-party payers) will be reading the plan of care to aid in their decision making regarding the patient. In the Assessment section, the PT assigns clinical meaning, or value, to the data collected during the examination process and, in the Plan section, the PT describes what he or she plans to do to help with the patient's problems. All information documented in this section of the note is substantiated by data collected in the examination and documented in the Subjective and Objective sections. To construct the Assessment and Plan, the PT uses sentences, paragraphs, and lists to give his or her impression of the patient and "tell the patient's story." The Assessment and Plan, or plan of care, include the following specific pieces of information.

Summary Statement, Diagnosis, and Problem List

Summary Statement

The Assessment section begins with the patient summary. This consists of a brief statement, or set of statements, that describe the patient (ie, age, gender, medical diagnosis). It answers the questions, "Who is this patient?" and "What is wrong with him or her?" The summary often includes a patient's medical diagnosis. The medical diagnosis comes from the patient's referral, the medical record, or even from the patient. In a direct access situation, the PT might indicate the medical diagnosis although there is debate on whether a PT should assign a medical diagnosis. The medical diagnosis is often the patient's pathology, disease, injury, or illness, such as multiple sclerosis, spinal cord injury, or humerus fracture. It may also include the relevant ICD-9 code(s).

Example 9-1. Example Summary Statements

A: 69-year-old female admitted 2 days ago after fall down stairs sustaining a right femur fracture; now 1 day status post-pinning.

A: 8-year-old female with myelomeningocele at the L1-2 level status post-recent growth spurt and functional decline.

A: 17-year-old female 2 weeks status post-grade 3 right ankle sprain.

Physical Therapy Diagnosis

The Assessment section also includes a physical therapy diagnosis. This is a diagnosis of the patient's movement disorders or dysfunction, and it describes the impact of an injury or condition on function at the systems level (especially the movement system) and at the whole-person level.[1] A diagnosis in this case is "both a process and a label."[1] Diagnosis as a "process" includes integrating and explaining relevant data obtained during the examination

and describing the patient/client condition in terms that will guide the prognosis and interventions.[1] The diagnostic "label" is the movement-related problem(s) that will also be addressed within the Plan section. To document the physical therapy diagnosis, provide a statement(s) that describe the relationship between the patient's impairments (identified in the exam data) and his or her activity limitations and participation restrictions (movement dysfunction). Also, document potential disabilities that may result if the impairments and functional deficits are not addressed appropriately. Use an appropriate heading (eg, PT diagnosis) when documenting the physical therapy diagnosis so that it is not confused with the medical diagnosis. The *Guide to Physical Therapist Practice* includes Preferred Practice Patterns in 4 body systems (musculoskeletal, neuromuscular, cardiovascular/pulmonary, and integumentary) that may serve as diagnostic categories (Appendix B). Alternatively, you may also choose to describe the movement dysfunction in your own words rather than using a guide-based category.

In this example, note how the impairments (decreased range of motion, strength, and mobility), all identified on the exam, have been linked to the patient's specific functional problems (ambulation, transfers, return to independent living, etc).

In these 2 latter examples, note how practice patterns from the *Guide to Physical Therapist Practice* were integrated and then linked to the patient's specific functional problems.

Example 9-2. Example of PT Diagnoses

A: 69-year-old woman admitted 2 days ago after fall down stairs sustaining a right femur fracture; now 1 day status post-pinning. PT Diagnosis: Decreased range of motion, strength, and weight bearing limiting the patient's ability to ambulate, transfer, and return to independent living, self-care, driving, and home management tasks.

A: 8-year-old girl with myelomeningocele at the L1-2 level status post-recent growth spurt and functional decline. PT Diagnosis: Impaired motor function and sensory integrity associated with nonprogressive disorders of the central nervous system limiting patient's ability to ambulate independently in the home, school, or community and perform independent self-care and transfers; puts patient at risk for skin breakdown.

A: 17-year-old girl 2 weeks status post-right bimalleolar fracture. PT Diagnosis: Impaired joint mobility, motor function, muscle performance, and range of motion associated with fracture limiting independent home, school, and community ambulation, driving, and participation in recreational activities.

Physical Therapy Problem List

In this section, the PT provides a list of specific physical therapy problems that will be addressed with the intervention. A problem list often includes some impairments, but the majority of problems should focus on patient-specific activity limitations and participation restrictions that were identified during the examination. To create the problem list, the PT looks back through the examination data and identifies relevant patient complaints and functional deficits given in the Subjective section, as well as abnormal results from tests and measures outlined in the Objective section, and records them in a list format. The problem list adds more detailed information to the PT diagnosis and it serves as a framework to create the latter sections of the Assessment and Plan.

Example 9-3. PT Problem List 1

A: 69-year-old woman admitted 2 days ago after fall down stairs sustaining a right femur fracture; now 1 day status post-pinning. <u>PT Diagnosis</u>: Decreased range of motion, strength, and weight bearing limiting the patient's ability to ambulate, transfer, and return to independent living, self-care, driving, and home management tasks. <u>Problem list</u>: 1) decreased hip and knee active range of motion; 2) decreased strength in the right lower extremity; 3) decreased ability to bear weight in the right lower extremity causing impaired balance; 4) dependent with bed and chair transfers; 5) dependent with sit to stand; 6) unable to ambulate without assistance; 7) unable to ascend and descend stairs; 8) unable to perform independent self-care, home management, or drive.

There may be times when the PT chooses to integrate the PT diagnosis and the problems list. In doing so, the problems are listed in a manner that relates a specific impairment to a specific activity limitation or participation restriction. One benefit of this is that it maintains the focus of the problem list on patient-specific function.

Example 9-4. PT Problem List 2

A: 8-year-old girl with myelomeningocele at the L1-2 level status post-recent growth spurt and functional decline. <u>PT Diagnosis and Problem List</u>: 1) Impaired motor function limiting the patient's ability to independently ambulate in her home, school, or community; 2) impaired motor function limiting patient's ability to perform independent self-care and transfers; 3) impaired sensory integrity making patient at risk for skin breakdown.

THE PATIENT'S PROGNOSIS

The Assessment section also includes the patient's prognosis. There are 3 components to the prognosis: (1) a statement regarding the patient's potential to benefit from the rehabilitation program, (2) a statement regarding problems or issues that may influence the intervention or the progress,

and (3) a list of outcome goals showing the "intended results" of the physical therapy interventions. Goals also include a specific target date for when they will be achieved.

Rehabilitation Potential

In many cases, the PT uses the terms *excellent*, *good*, *fair*, or *poor* to document a patient's rehabilitation potential. Although documenting potential in this manner is fairly common in clinical practice, there are no well-established criteria that constitute excellent, good, fair, or poor potential. In addition, authors have shown that this method is not reliable between different therapists.[4] When using this terminology to describe rehabilitation potential, it seems that if the PT has considered all the necessary factors and set appropriate goals and time frames, then the patient's potential to meet the established goals should be good. If the potential is poor, then the PT should reconsider whether the patient is appropriate for therapy services or reconsider the established goals.

Factors That May Influence the Intervention, Progress, or Outcome

In addition, the PT considers and documents any issues that might influence the intervention plan and recovery time. These issues include (1) comorbidities, or concomitant diagnoses unrelated to the treating diagnosis (eg, a patient with a hip fracture also has chronic obstructive pulmonary disease); (2) complexities, a concomitant diagnosis that is related to the treating diagnosis (eg, a patient with rheumatoid arthritis undergoes a total shoulder replacement); or (3) complicating factors, issues that arise from the original diagnosis (eg, a postsurgical infection). The PT also considers and documents any other issues (eg, cognitive, psychological, social, economic) that might complicate or slow down the rehabilitative process. This information can be combined with the rehabilitation potential to provide a better picture of the therapist's expectations.

Example 9-5. Rehab Potential Examples

1. The patient's potential to benefit from therapy and achieve the goals stated is excellent because of his excellent motivation and health status.
2. The patient's potential to benefit from the intervention is good. Time since injury may influence how quickly the patient may recover.
3. The patient has good potential to achieve the goals established; however, his medical history, including diabetes and congestive heart failure, may influence length of recovery.
4. The patient has good potential to achieve the established goals; however, chronic wound on the sound limb will interfere with gait training.

Anticipated Goals and Expected Outcomes

The prognosis includes a list of goals or expected outcomes written to reflect the patient's final status at the end of the episode of care. They may be called outcome goals, expected outcomes, discharge goals, or long-term goals (LTGs). When writing a goal, the PT determines the anticipated level of improvement based on the data and knowledge of the condition and the time required to reach this level. Perfecting goal-writing skills requires practice and seeing patient progression in a variety of circumstances helps in this process. An important thing to remember is that any component of the prognosis, including the outcome goals, may be modified at any point in the episode of care if the patient is progressing faster or slower than what was expected. A statement(s) that provides a justification for revising goals is included.

The Mechanics of Goal Writing

Well-written goals include 4 parts. As a guide, remember the ABCD of goal writing. "A" stands for *audience*, this is the individual who will be demonstrating the behavior or the attribute. In physical therapy, the "A" should be the patient or the patient's family member or caregiver. The "A" is *not* the therapist or another health care provider. "B" stands for *behavior*. The behavior is the action or attribute(s) being performed or assessed. A behavior might be a functional task such as walking, getting in or out of bed, or reaching. It might be learned information such as hip precautions. A behavior might be a specific attribute the patient displays such as muscle strength, blood pressure, or pain. "C" stands for *condition*. This includes a description of the conditions under which the behavior is to be performed. Conditions could include the environmental setting in which the behavior will be performed (eg, on level surfaces) or the presence or absence of assistive or adaptive equipment. "D" stands for *degree*. This is the degree to which the attribute should be demonstrated. This is a measurable term. A degree might be the specific muscle grade that is expected, the level of assist needed, the time it will take to complete a task, or the degree of accuracy that is expected.

The acronym SMART is also used to describe an appropriately structured goal. SMART stands for *specific, measurable, attainable, realistic,* and *timely*. This acronym incorporates many of the components as outlined in the ABCD method, but it also highlights the concept of making sure the goals are attainable and realistic. This is important when the patient's prognosis is difficult to determine because of the complexity of the problems.

Example 9-6. Sample Goals

1. In 6 weeks, the patient will demonstrate increased active hip extension to 20 degrees to allow normal prosthetic gait.

---

2. In 3 months, the patient's strength will increase from 2/5 to 4/5 to increase independence with sit to stand, transfers, and safe ambulation.

3. In 6 visits, the patient's pain will decrease from 9/10 to 4/10 to allow patient to achieve a full night of sleep.

Whether you are using the ABCD or SMART method, goals should always be specific and measurable to allow for ease in outcomes assessment, and they should paint a very clear picture of what the patient will look like at the end of the episode of care. As a rule of thumb, write a goal for every problem identified in the problem list (Example 9-7). Take note, however, that a single goal can be written to include multiple problems. When writing goals, one can address impairments, activity limitations, and/or participation restrictions. But, when writing a goal at the impairment level, relate it to a functional activity that will also be improved as the impairment is resolved.

Example 9-7. Example Assessment

A: 59-y.o. man s/p fall at work sustaining a (R) rotator cuff tear 6 months ago; now 1 week following repair (ICD-9 840.4); PT diagnosis is impaired joint mobility, motor function, muscle performance, and ROM due to connective tissue dysfunction (Practice Pattern 4D) limiting his ability to elevate arm overhead, reach overhead cabinets, perform normal home management tasks, or perform work activities as a custodian. Pt. has type 2 diabetes that may slow progress but pt. reports motivation to return to work.

PT Problems
*Impairments**
   a. Pain at rest and with activity
   b. Decreased ROM
   c. Decreased strength
   d. Healing surgical incision with ecchymosis

Activity Limitations and Participation Restrictions
   a. Moderate to severe difficulty on ADL
   b. Unable to elevate arm overhead
   c. Severe difficulty sleeping due to pain
   d. Unable to manage transportation needs
   e. Unable to work
   f. Unable to participate in recreational activities
   g. DASH score 55/100

The patient demonstrates good potential for full recovery and to meet PT goals. In 16 weeks, the patient will demonstrate:

   a. Pain < 3/10 to allow a full night's sleep[†]
   b. 165 degrees of shoulder flexion to allow full arm elevation to perform overhead activities[†]

c. Strength in the shoulder girdle muscles 4/5 to allow full use upon RTW[†]

d. Healed surgical scar with no complications

e. Independent with and pain free ADL

f. Independent in managing transportation needs

g. Return to work with minimal to no limitations

h. Full participation in recreational activities

i. Final DASH score < 20

*The problem list can be broken down as shown here or one list may be created.

[†]Note how this goal includes an impairment but it is related to function. It also addresses two problems from the problem list.

Integrating the Evidence Into Goal Writing

In recent literature, authors have suggested several methods to incorporate the evidence on an instrument's measurement properties into patient goals.[5,6] For example, a goal may reflect a value that would be considered "normal" for a particular test or measure. Goals may include relevant properties such as the instrument's minimal detectable change (MDC) or the minimal clinically important difference (MCID). These values provide the amount of change that would be clinically relevant or clinically meaningful to the patient, respectively. Goals may include values that discriminate one population from another (eg, Berg Balance Score of 45 is indicative of fall risk)[7] or that coincide with a specific level of disability.[5] When specific values of an instrument are not known, the goal may be written so that the degree of change exceeds the instrument's associated amount of error at minimum. One may also choose to examine prognostic studies for establishing an appropriate benchmark for a patient's goals. Using measurement properties in this manner requires the PT to be familiar with the current literature regarding the tests and measures used clinically and it integrates evidence into practice.

MacDermid and Stratford[5] provided an example of a patient with rotator cuff disease. During an initial examination, a patient's score on the DASH self-report questionnaire was 44. In deciding goals for this patient, the PT was also able to extrapolate from the literature that an MCID on the DASH is approximately 15 points. Therefore, he wrote the following outcome goal for the patient[5]:

In 12 weeks, the patient will demonstrate an important change in his DASH score (> 15 points).

The PT knew from Beaton et al[8] that a score of 26.8 on the DASH coincided with a patient returning to work.[5] So the following goal was written:

In 3 months, the patient will demonstrate a DASH score < 25.

In this example, the PT used the value reported in the literature that discriminates patients who are working versus those who are not. This could accompany a goal for the patient to return to work. Using the tool's measurement properties can help write goals and reflect meaningful clinical changes in a patient's status. In an ideal world, data on measurement tools would be easily available to clinicians; however, this is usually not the case and clinicians may have to extrapolate from more general research findings.[5] Using measurement properties in documentation is discussed further in later chapters.

Establishing the Goal's Time Frame

The time it takes to reach the outcome goals is a clinical judgment made by the PT. The time frame is set in terms of days, visits, weeks, or months. One important factor for consideration is the medical diagnosis. For example, the expectations for recovery are very different for a patient with a minor musculoskeletal condition versus one with a degenerative neuromuscular disorder. Other considerations include the particular setting, rehabilitation protocol, and time for tissue healing to occur. For example, a patient is recovering from a cerebrovascular accident and is receiving physical therapy services in an inpatient rehabilitation hospital. The PT chooses to set the time frame on the outcome goals based on how long he suspects the patient will be in the unit (eg, 2 weeks). In another example, a patient undergoes an Achilles tendon repair, the PT examines the patient and, based on the established protocol and time for tissue healing, sets the time frame for 12 to 16 weeks. The following are examples of goals that are suitable for documentation in a patient's medical record.

Example 9-8. Sample Goals

1. In 3 days, the patient will ambulate 50' with a standard walker 50% weight bearing on the left lower extremity with close supervision on level surfaces

2. In 6 weeks the patient will show increased shoulder flexion from 90 to 165 degrees to allow improved overhead reaching.

3. In 3 weeks the patient will demonstrate normal vital signs after ambulating with supervision for 500'.

4. In 12 weeks the patient's Berg Balance Test will increase to 50 indicating no longer at risk for falling.[7]

5. In 3 weeks the patient's husband will be independent with assisting the patient during car transfers.

6. In 6 weeks the patient's quadriceps strength will increase from 3/5 to 4+/5 to allow improved ability to rise from the floor and stair climbing.

7. In 2 weeks the child will be able to hold her head at midline while focusing on a toy for 1 minute.

8. In 3 days the patient will transfer from the bed to and from the wheelchair with minimal assist during sit to stand and to maintain weight-bearing precautions.

9. In 30 days the patient will be independent with home ambulation (~250') with a straight cane on carpet and hard surfaces.

10. The infant will bring both hands to midline without prompting in 6 weeks.

11. In 10 visits the patient will be able to have full finger range of motion to allow full grip during home tasks and recreational activities.

12. In 4 weeks the patient will ambulate 500' on a variety of surfaces with a quad cane and supervision with a velocity exceeding 1.0 m/s.

13. In 6 weeks the patient's Fugl-Meyer Upper Extremity score will improve 8% to 10%.[9]

14. In 4 weeks the patient's score on the Foot and Ankle Ability measure will increase 8-10 points.[6,10]

15. In 6 weeks the patient's score on the Penn Shoulder Scale will increase 15 points.[11]

Short-Term Goals

If there is a significant difference between the patient's current condition and the expected outcomes (outcome goals), the therapist may choose to include STGs. STGs serve as "bridge" goals between the patient's current status and the long-term expected outcome goals. Any STG written generally reflects a long-term, outcome goal. However, not all outcome goals have STGs and vice versa. STGs are desirable for several reasons. One reason is to help guide the decision-making process. As the patient progresses through the episode of care, STGs are used as landmarks or stepping stones to help the therapist determine if the patient is making the desired/expected progress within a reasonable amount of time. Without STGs, it can be more difficult for the therapist to gauge if the patient is making satisfactory progress. STGs also provide an excellent recording mechanism for third-party payers to demonstrate the patient's response to the physical therapy plan of care. Third-party payers demand documentation that interventions are influencing the patient's problem(s), and STGs are a useful method to allow clear communication of the patient's progress. Finally, STGs provide a motivating factor for the patient. During a long-term rehabilitative process, patients can often become discouraged with what seems like little to no change from day to day, but STGs can provide small but realistic expectations and stepping stones on which the patient can focus. Look at the following examples.

Example 9-9. Short-Term Goals

1. The patient will ambulate 50' with a standard walker 50% weight bearing on the left lower extremity with close supervision on level surfaces.

   STG: The patient will ambulate 25' with a standard walker non-weight bearing on the left lower extremity with minimal assist of one for sequencing and balance in single-limb stance.

2. The patient will show increased shoulder flexion from 90 to 165 degrees to allow improved overhead reaching.

   STG: The patient will show increased shoulder flexion from 90 to 120 degrees to allow reaching into a low cabinet and improved ADL performance.

3. The patient will demonstrate normal vital signs after ambulating with supervision for 500'.

   STG: The patient will demonstrate normal vital signs after ambulating with contact guard assist of one for 100'.

THE INTERVENTION PLAN

The Amount, Frequency, and Duration

The Plan section delineates the amount, frequency, and duration of services that the patient will need to achieve the established goals and outcomes. In an inpatient setting, this might be twice daily for the next 3 to 4 days or 1 time daily, 5 times per week, for the next 4 weeks. In skilled nursing settings, it is important that the amount and frequency, or total therapy minutes, correspond with the patient's corresponding "RUG level." You will read more about this in later chapters. In an outpatient setting, this may read 3 times per week for 6 weeks or twice weekly for 3 months. Although some goals will be met sooner than others, in general, it is important that the duration of services provided in the plan matches the longest time frame written on the discharge goals. See the following example. *Plan duration cannot be longer than our LTG*

Example 9-10. Amount, Frequency, and Duration

Discharge goals:

1. The patient will demonstrate decreased pain from 7/10 to 2/10 in 4 weeks to allow pain-free ambulation.

2. The patient will be independent in all transfers in 8 weeks.

3. The patient will return home to live independently in 8 weeks.

Plan: The patient will be seen twice daily, 6 days per week, for the next 8 weeks.

The duration of services in this example matches the time frame set on goal 3, which is the time in which the PT thinks the patient will be discharged from the facility. Note the time frame on goal 1 is for 4 weeks. It is assumed that once this is achieved, the therapist will be working toward the other established goals.

Plan for Skilled Care

When using the SOAP format, the Plan section also includes a statement summarizing the plan for skilled services. This is a statement(s) that provides an overview of the therapist's skills the patient needs to achieve the desired outcomes. It serves as a general statement to indicate the skilled care to be provided and "sets the stage" for the more specific list of interventions that will follow. It is important to use the term "skilled services" in this section. Skills indicated in this aspect of the note can include education, safety, progression, etc. This is an area of documentation that is still emerging and often difficult to articulate. In using the SOAP structure, one may find this statement in the A aspect of the note. Look at the examples that follow to see how you can provide this important piece of information.

Example 9-11. Plans for Skilled Care

1. Skilled services will be provided to educate the patient on surgical precautions, assist in performing safe transfers, instruct and assist in weight-bearing precautions and use of assistive device, and provide a safe exercise progression to improve motion and strength.

2. Skilled services will be provided to design and implement safe activities to promote normal trunk and head alignment, to instruct the parents in proper handling skills to decrease tone, and to educate parents on adaptive seating.

Specific Services to Be Provided

The plan also includes a more detailed list of specific interventions that will be provided. This list includes the scientific rationale for providing the specific intervention(s) to show medical necessity. Interventions include procedural interventions and nonprocedural interventions, such as patient education and communication with other health care providers. Procedural interventions include techniques and procedures used by a PT or PTA (as directed by the PT) designed to impact the patient's condition in effort to achieve the goals and outcomes. Procedural interventions are the activities that most people consider when the term "physical therapy" is used. Procedural interventions fall in 9 categories outlined in the *Guide to Physical Therapist Practice*[1]: (1) therapeutic exercise; (2) functional training in self-care and home management; (3) functional training in work (job/school/play); (4) manual therapy techniques; (5) prescription, application, and (as appropriate) fabrication of devices and equipment; (6) airway clearance techniques; (7) integumentary repair and protective techniques; (8) electrotherapeutic modalities; and (9) physical agents and mechanical modalities. When documenting the procedural interventions, include enough detail to describe

what will be done and **why** it will be done; but, do not write it in a way that will require unnecessary frequent updates or modifications. For example, the PT might indicate that electrotherapeutic agents will be used to address pain but specific parameters do not necessarily need to be included. This will allow the therapist to choose between different devices and alter the parameters without the necessity of updating the plan of care each time.

The Plan section also outlines nonprocedural interventions such as coordination, communication, and/or collaboration with other health care providers along with a justification. "Coordination is the working together of all parties involved with the patient/client."[1] It is accomplished through various types of communication and documentation. Therefore, it is important to document any plans to consult with other care providers. For example, if during the examination process the PT determines that the patient's medication regimen is impacting the patient's responses negatively, he or she will document a plan to discuss these issues with the physician. As an autonomous practitioner, an important role of a PT is to collaborate with physicians, nurses, occupational therapists, and other health care providers. Often, individuals confuse the concept of "autonomous" mistakenly thinking it means that the PT acts in a totally independent, "Lone Ranger" method. Rather, the concept of "autonomous" indicates that the PT is entirely responsible for all aspects of physical therapy care. In order to accomplish that task, the PT needs to collaborate with the other members of the health care team. The PT has a unique and important perspective to share with the team, while at the same time having a responsibility to realize the limitations of that view. Therefore, the PT must have a high regard for the information and perspectives provided by other health care providers.

The importance of patient education within the intervention cannot be overstated. It is through the educational process that the patient and the patient's family or caregiver are assisted in taking full and complete ownership of the patient's health and well-being. Helping patients develop the knowledge, skills, and attitudinal framework necessary to manage their own health care concerns moves them to independence. Patient-related instruction can encompass several different topics, including education about (1) the pathology/disease process, (2) the body structure or body function impairments, (3) functional limitations, (4) how those impairments and functional limitations impact the patient's participation within social roles, (5) the physical therapy plan of care, (6) general health issues such as the patient's need for a fitness program or information regarding appropriate nutrition, (7) a home exercise program, (8) home or work modifications, (9) functional task training, (10) precautions or restrictions, and (11) appropriate activity level based on the pathology.[1(p47)] Within the plan, document specific topics and information that will be provided to a patient. For example, a patient who is recovering from a total hip arthroplasty will require targeted information related to hip arthroplasty precautions. Goals may be written that reflect specific aspects of patient education and that patient learning has occurred.

Example 9-12. Specific Planned Interventions and Rationale

Specific Interventions:

1. Hip and knee ther ex to improve ROM and strength to improve ambulation and transfers.
2. Gait training to improve home mobility, safety, and (I) living.
3. Transfer training to promote home independence and safety with weight-bearing restrictions.
4. Discuss home equipment needs with case manager.

In some instances, the plan may also state the date of the next formal reassessment or reevaluation and give the discharge plan(s). Discharge plans may include transfer to another setting for further physical therapy services (eg, transfer from acute care hospital to a skilled nursing facility) or discharge to a home maintenance program (Example 9-13).

Example 9-13. Example Plan 1

P: The patient will be seen 2× per week for the next 12-16 weeks. Skilled care will be provided to educate patient on precautions, safe progression of therapeutic exercises, appropriate use of sling and abduction pillow, and to educate spouse on assistance during home exercises. For the next 5 weeks, the patient will receive 1) passive range of motion to improve flexion, abduction, IR, and ER to allow full capsular mobility and prevent adhesive capsulitis since the patient is at risk because of diabetes; 2) modalities to control pain; 3) active scapular exercises to promote scapulothoracic mobility; and 4) instruction in a home exercise program. In 6 weeks there will be a reassessment to determine the appropriate interventions at that time that will allow him to meet the above goals and return to his prior status including RTW.

HOW A PHYSICAL THERAPIST ASSISTANT USES THE ASSESSMENT AND PLAN (PLAN OF CARE)

The diagnosis, prognosis, and intervention plan, documented within the Assessment and Plan sections of the SOAP note, are of vital importance for the PTA. The PTA reviews the assessment to find out the reason for therapy services, the specific problems to be addressed, issues that may influence the intervention, and the anticipated goals. The PTA reviews the plan to identify the interventions

that will be provided. The Plan section is of particular importance because it provides the guideline(s) for the interventions the PTA can legally perform. For example, a PT directs the assistant to work with a patient on functional mobility. The assistant reviews the Assessment section to understand the patient's diagnosis, mobility problems, and prognosis. This will help the assistant have appropriate and realistic expectations and be able to anticipate the patient's responses to the interventions. The PTA references the plan to determine specific mobility skills to address and parameters in which he or she can legally progress the patient since the PTA can adjust the interventions only within the guidelines documented with the plan. The PTA also references the plan when he or she feels that a patient's interventions should be adjusted. Look at the following example.

Example 9-14. Example Plan 2

P: Skilled services will be provided to educate the patient on use of a standard walker, provide cueing during ambulation for safety and weight-bearing precautions, and to perform range of motion exercises to improve knee and hip mobility allowing the patient to ascend and descend stairs and sit comfortably. The patient will also receive functional mobility training to improve safety and independence so that she can return to living independently at home. Pt will be seen 2x/day for 3 to 5 days.

In this example, the PT has identified the assistive device, interventions, and functional training that this patient will receive. If this were a real plan, then a PTA could *not* advance the assistive device to a cane and the PTA could *not* perform strengthening exercises because these are not part of the established plan. A PTA could, however, choose the range of motion exercises and the mobility training since these are less prescriptive. As you can see, the amount of detail provided in a plan determines how the PTA can progress the patient. Also, if the patient is not responding to the established plan, the PTA communicates with the PT and suggests possible changes to the plan. Or, if the patient is responding quickly and the PTA feels the patient should have more advanced exercises or intervention, again, there is communication to the PT for plan adjustments.

When reviewing the Assessment and Plan sections of the SOAP note, the assistant will have the following questions in mind[12]:

- What interventions does the PT want me to provide?
- What problem(s) is the intervention addressing?
- What are the goals for this patient?
- What is the patient's diagnosis?
- What is the patient's prognosis?
- Are there any contraindications or precautions I need to keep in mind?
- Are there any other special issues I need to keep in mind?

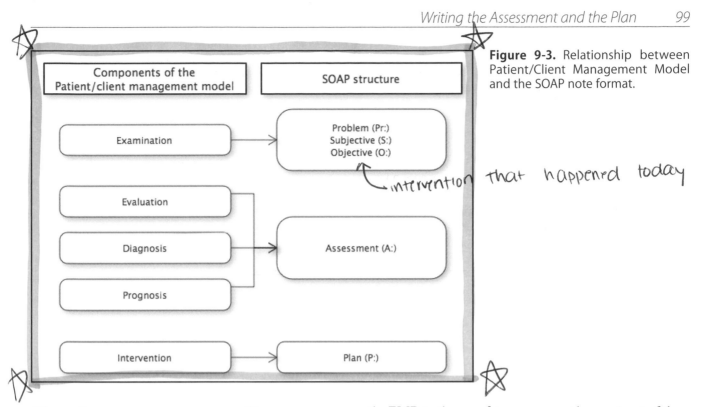

Figure 9-3. Relationship between Patient/Client Management Model and the SOAP note format.

THE ASSESSMENT AND PLAN IN AN ELECTRONIC MEDICAL RECORD

Templates of a physical therapy EMR often consist of a series of drop-down menus and check boxes to facilitate ease of documentation. There are often templates for many aspects of the Assessment and Plan sections, or plan of care. There may be a list of choices for establishing the problem list; check boxes for rehabilitation potential; check boxes for factors that influence treatment; a list of preestablished goals; check boxes for the interventions to be provided; as well as check boxes for the amount, frequency, and duration of services. When documenting using predetermined lists or choices in this manner, it is easy to rapidly over-select or get into a habit of selecting the same choices for all patients. This, along with the "canned" phrases generated by some software programs, can quickly limit the individual nature of the problem list and often does not reflect a patient's unique problems, functional demands, and lifestyle. In addition, it is difficult to articulate the need for skilled care and medical necessity of the interventions using predetermined check boxes and lists. With the need for health care providers to transition to the EMR in the near future, one must be cognizant of these issues and create documentation that includes necessary components of contemporary documentation, captures a patient's unique status and needs, and maintains patient individuality within the diagnosis, problems list, goals, and interventions.

SUMMARY

At the onset of physical therapy services, it is imperative that documentation outlines the findings from the examination and evaluation and includes a detailed plan of care. The SOAP note is a common documentation format that can be used for this process. The SOAP format outlines the findings from the examination in the Subjective and Objective sections and details the evaluation, diagnosis, prognosis, and interventions within the Assessment and Plan sections (Figure 9-3). This initial documentation provides the format and foundational information on which all future physical therapy sessions are based. All future documentation should refer to the structure and information provided within the initial note (see Figure 9-2; see also Figures 4-1, 5-3, and 5-4).

REVIEW QUESTIONS

1. List the information that is found within the Assessment and Plan sections of the SOAP note.
Summary Statement, PT diagnosis, Problem list, rehab potential, Plan for Skilled care, frequency, duration

2. Describe the relationship between the examination and the evaluation.

3. Differentiate between a linear clinical decision-making model and a dynamic clinical decision-making model. Which model best describes the process that is often used within the physical therapy evaluative process?

4. Differentiate between the medical diagnosis and the physical therapy diagnosis.

the PT diagnosis is a description of how the injury (medical diagnosis) impacts movement

5. How should the PT construct a physical therapy diagnosis?

describe the relationship between the patient's impairments and their activity limitations

6. List some considerations for developing a prognosis.

potential to benefit from rehab program, problems that may interfere w/ interventions, outcome goals

7. List and describe the components of a well-written goal.

A - Audence   C - condition
B - Behavior   D - degree ← measurable

8. How can a PT integrate evidence regarding tests and measures into goal statements?

9. How does the PTA use the information documented in the Assessment and Plan sections of a SOAP note? How can the therapist structure the note to enhance the PT/PTA relationship?

10. Outline an appropriate structure for the documentation of the Assessment and Plan sections of a SOAP note.

APPLICATION EXERCISES

1. Read the following goals and identify the audience, behavior, condition, and degree. Also identify components that are missing. When appropriate, determine if the goal addresses an impairment, an activity limitation, or a participation restriction.

   a. STG: Decreased turgor and fibrosis by 50% (to a 7 × 15 cm area) within 4 to 6 visits.

   b. STG: Decrease girth of (R) ankle to within 1 cm of (L) (using figure 8) in 3 visits.

   c. LTG: The patient will demonstrate mastery of pacing and other overuse reduction strategies to allow him to return to work.

   d. STG: Decrease pain to 3/10 during movement.

   e. LTG: Patient will display normal gait pattern.

   f. LTG: In 4 to 6 weeks, the patient will be (I) with bed mobility & transfers including supine to and from sit; w/c to and from bed (no sliding board); and w/c to and from floor.

   g. LTG: In 4 to 6 weeks, the patient will be (I) with w/c mobility on level surfaces, up and down curbs, and on uneven surfaces.

   h. STG: The patient will verbalize 3/3 hip precautions without verbal prompts.

   i. LTG: In 8 weeks, the patient will participate in a community outing with only min (A) of 1.

   j. STG: The wound will have an area of 2 × 2 cm with 1 cm depth.

2. Match the appropriate short-term goal for the following outcome goals.

3. Given the following data provided in an initial examination, write a goal if the expectation is that the patient will improve.

Outcome goal	Short-term goals (STGs)
1. The patient will ambulate with prosthesis 500' without assistive device on varied terrain with close supervision in 6 weeks.	A. The patient will manage his wheelchair on a variety of surfaces 250' with minimal verbal cueing in 2 weeks.
2. The patient will transfer to and from all surfaces with supervision in 2 weeks.	B. The patient will transfer to and from the right independently and to and from the left with minimal assist of one in 3 to 5 days.
3. The patient will manage his wheelchair independently for 500' in an open environment to allow independent community mobility in 1 month.	C. The patient will ambulate 75' with a standard walker and the prosthesis with minimal assist of 1 for balance and weight shifting in 3 weeks.

_G_ 4. The patient will ambulate 150' with prosthesis and standard walker on level surfaces independently in 6 weeks.	D. The patient will propel his wheelchair on level surfaces 50-75' with verbal cues in 2 weeks.
_D_ 5. The patient will manage his wheelchair 100' on level surfaces and small inclines independently in 4 weeks.	E. The patient will ambulate 250' with prosthesis and quad cane on level surfaces and small inclines with supervision and verbal cues in 3 weeks.

    a. <u>Strength</u>: 5/5 throughout (B) LEs except (R) quadriceps 3/5 because of pain and (R) hamstrings 3/5 because of disuse.

    b. <u>AROM</u>   <u>Left</u>   <u>Right</u>

	Left	Right
1. DF	0 to 20 degrees	−5 degrees from neutral
2. PF	0 to 40 degrees	5 degrees

    c. <u>Mobility</u>: Bed mobility: rolling with mod (A) × 1 and frequent verbal cues for sequencing and set up.

    d. <u>Transfers</u>: Bed/mat to and from w/c with max (A) of 1 to 2, dependent with all set up

    e. <u>Gait</u>: Pt. ambulated 50' with small-based quad cane and mod (A) × 1 to assist with upright posture and increasing step length. Pt. displayed ataxia, motor planning, and motor sequencing deficits.

4. Review the following information, and using the *Guide to Physical Therapist Practice*, identify an appropriate practice pattern that matches the description given.

    a. The patient entered physical therapy through self-referral. The patient's primary complaint is back pain. The patient demonstrates a flattening of the lumbar spine, increased kyphosis of the thoracic spine, a forward head, and rounded shoulder posturing.

    b. The patient underwent an open reduction and internal fixation for a hip fracture. The patient has pain, decreased range of motion, decreased strength, and decreased mobility.

    c. The patient is 7 years old and has a diagnosis of cerebral palsy. The patient demonstrates delayed motor development, abnormal postural reflex responses, difficulties with communication, and delayed cognitive development.

    d. This client participated in a community outreach health risk appraisal held at a local community center. The individual denied any history of medical problems other than hypertension. The individual reported a maternal history of stroke and a paternal history of heart disease. The patient was mildly obese.

    e. This patient sustained burns to both hands while burning leaves in his yard. The burns were partial thickness burns.

5. Review the Assessment and Plan sections of the note as found in Example 9-15. Critique the note using the following questions.

    a. Does the note provide a physical therapy diagnosis? *NO*

    b. Does the note clearly demonstrate the clinical decision-making process? *NO*

    c. Does the note draw correlations between information about impairment and function? *NO*

    d. Does the note demonstrate the relationship between the problem list, the goals, and the interventions? *yes NO*

    e. Are the interventions clearly detailed to guide the PTA? *NO*

6. Example 9-16 is the initial subjective and objective documentation for a patient recently admitted to an acute care hospital. Use it to help you complete the Assessment and Plan sections of the note.

Example 9-15. Example Assessment and Plan from Initial Documentation

Assessment:

59-y.o. woman 2 weeks s/p fall injuring right knee and development of pneumonia; hospitalized × 5 days

Problem List

1. Knee pain
2. Limited ROM
3. Limited strength
4. Gait disturbance

<u>STGs</u>, 2 weeks

1. Decrease pain
2. Increase strength by one full grade
3. Increase AROM, PROM, and hamstring length by 20 degrees and gastroc 10 degrees
4. WNL gait pattern

LTGs: Resume maximum function of the (L) knee and discharge to home

Plan: PT bid for ROM and gait until discharge. Add strengthening exercises when pain decreases.

REFERENCES

1. American Physical Therapy Association. *Guide to Physical Therapist Practice.* 2nd ed. Alexandria, VA: APTA; 2003.
2. Jones MA. Clinical reasoning in manual therapy. *Phys Ther.* 1992;72:43-52.
3. Centers for Medicare & Medicaid Services. Covered medical and other health services. *Medicare Benefit Policy Manual.* Publication 100-02. http://www.cms.gov/Regulations-and-Guidance/Guidance/Manuals/Downloads/bp102c15.pdf. Accessed May 16, 2012.
4. Cunningham C, Horgan F, O'Neill D. Clinical assessment of rehabilitation potential of the older patient: a pilot study. *Clin Rehabil.* 2000;14:205-207.
5. MacDermid JC, Stratford P. Applying evidence on outcome measures to hand therapy practice. *J Hand Ther.* 2004;17:165-173.
6. Martin RL, Irrgang JJ, Burdett RG, Conti SF, Van Swearingen JM. Evidence of validity for the Foot and Ankle Ability Measure. *Foot & Ankle Int.* 2006;26:968-983.
7. Riddle DL, Stratford PW. Interpreting validity indexes for diagnostic tests: an illustration using the Berg Balance Test. *Phys Ther.* 1999;79:939-948.

Example 9-16. Example Subjective and Objective Sections of SOAP Note

Initial Evaluation

Date: 08/10/12

Pr: (L) CVA, (R) hemiplegia; <u>HPI</u>: 67 y.o. male was admitted to the acute care 08/08/12 because of sudden weakness in his (R) UE & LE and slurred speech. <u>PMH</u>: NIDDM, HTN, CABG × 2 07/05/2005. Height: 6' 2" Weight: 255#; No other pertinent medical history. Current medications include glucophage and captopril.

S: <u>C/C</u>: Inability to move, function, care for himself; weakness in (R) UE & LE; pain in the (R) shoulder 5/10. <u>Prior level of function</u>: (I) with all ADL, IADL, and gait without an assistive device. Active; worked in his woodshop, yard, and garden; performed all necessary home management tasks. He is (R) hand dominant. <u>Home situation</u>: Retired carpenter; lives with his wife who is healthy but is a small woman. Lives in 2-level home with 4 steps to enter. <u>Patient's goals</u>: Return to prior lifestyle.

O: *Systems Review:* <u>CP System</u>: HR, 96 bpm; BP, 128/88; RR, 14. <u>Integumentary system</u>: Not impaired. <u>Cognition/Communication</u>: Slurred speech. Alert and oriented × 4.

Tests/Measures: <u>Observation</u>: 3+ pitting edema in (R) hand and forearm; tendency to keep (R) UE in dependent position. <u>Figure 8 hand girth</u>: (R) 54 cm, (L) 52. cm. <u>Capillary refill</u>: Normal. <u>Sensation</u>: Diminished light touch, deep pressure localization, proprioception & kinesthesia through the (R) UE & LE. <u>Muscle Tone</u>: diminished tone on (R) UE & LE to passive range. <u>Reflexes</u>: diminished patellar reflexes and absent Achilles reflex on (R). <u>Shoulder</u>: 1 finger width sulcus at (R) GH joint. <u>Balance</u>: Unable to stand without physical assistance or UE support. <u>Endurance</u>: Pt. tolerated 30-minute session requiring 1-minute rest breaks every 5-8 minutes. <u>Posture</u>: Trunk in laterally flexed position and slightly rotated to the left. <u>Strength</u>:

	<u>Right</u>	<u>Left</u>
Shoulder		
Flexion	2-/5	5/5
Extension	2-/5	5/5
Abduction	2-/5	5/5
IR/ER	2-/5	5/5
Elbow		
Flexion	2-/5	5/5
Extension	2-/5	5/5
Wrist		
Flexion	2-/5	5/5
Extension	2-/5	5/5
Finger		
Flexion	1/5	5/5
Hip		
Flexion	3-/5	5/5
Extension	3-/5	5/5
Abduction	3+/5	5/5
Adduction	3+/5	5/5
IR	3+/5	5/5
ER	3+/5	5/5
Knee		
Flexion	3+/5	5/5
Extension	3-/5	5/5
Ankle		
DF	2-/5	5/5
PF	2-/5	5/5

Functional Status: <u>Bed Mobility</u>: Max(a) × 1 scooting up/down and side/side in bed; mod (a) × 1 rolling to (L); min (a) × 1 rolling to (R) <u>Transfers</u>: Supine ↔ sit min (a) × 1 from (R) side and mod (a) × 1 from (L) side; sit ↔ stand mod (a) × 2; stand pivot w/c ↔ bed mod (A) × 2. <u>Gait</u>: ambulated in // × 8' × 2 with mod (a) × 2; Reqd. 1 to stabilize and balance at the trunk and 1 for assisting with advancing the (R) LE and stabilizing the (R) UE; Reqd. verbal cues for sequencing as patient very impulsive during gait. <u>W/C management</u>: Dependent in parts and mobility.

8. Beaton DE, Katz JN, Fossel AH, Wright JG, Tarasuk V. Measuring the whole or parts: validity, reliability, and responsiveness of the DASH outcome measure in different regions of the upper extremity. *J Hand Ther.* 2001;14:128-146.

9. Page SJ, Fulk GD, Boyne P. Clinically important differences for the Upper-Extremity Fugl-Meyer Scale in people with minimal to moderate impairment due to chronic stroke. *Phys Ther.* 2012;92:791-798.

10. Martin RL, Irrgang JJ. A survey of self-reported outcome instruments for the foot and ankle. *J Orthop Sports Phys Ther.* 2007;37:72-84.

11. Leggin BG, Michener LA, Shaffer MA, Brenneman SK, Iannotti JP, Williams GW. The Penn Shoulder Score: reliability and validity. *J Orthop Sports Phys Ther.* 2006;36:138-151.

12. Erickson ML, McKnight R. *Documentation Basics: A Guide for the PTA.* 2nd ed. Thorofare, NJ: SLACK Incorporated; 2012.

Chapter 10

Interim Documentation

Mia L. Erickson, PT, EdD, CHT, ATC and Rebecca McKnight, PT, MS

CHAPTER OUTLINE

CHAPTER OBJECTIVES

Upon completion of this chapter, the reader will be able to:
1. Describe types of documentation that occur across the episode of care.
2. List the various types of interim documentation.
3. Discuss the roles of the PT and the PTA in documenting interim notes.
4. Differentiate between a treatment note and a progress note.
5. Document the intervention aspect of an interim note.
6. Identify factors that would indicate the need for a reevaluation.
7. Discuss the relationship between the initial documentation and interim notes.
8. Describe the contents of a letter to a physician.
9. Integrate evidence in clinical decision making when examining patient change.
10. Construct a progress note.

Erickson ML, Utzman RR, McKnight R. *Physical Therapy Documentation:*
From Examination to Outcome, Second Edition (pp 105-115).
© 2014 SLACK Incorporated.

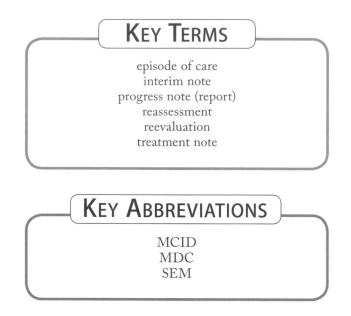

KEY TERMS

episode of care
interim note
progress note (report)
reassessment
reevaluation
treatment note

KEY ABBREVIATIONS

MCID
MDC
SEM

Physical therapy documentation occurs over the patient's entire episode of care. The physical therapy record clearly describes (1) the patient's condition, or pathology; (2) impairments in body structures and body functions; (3) functional or activity limitations and participation restrictions; (4) the PT's clinical reasoning and rationale; (5) anticipated goals and expected outcomes; (6) skilled interventions provided, including patient education, communication with other disciplines, and specific procedural interventions; and (7) the final outcome, or result of the intervention.

APTA's *Guidelines for Physical Therapy Documentation of Patient/Client Management* indicates that documentation is required for every patient visit/encounter.[1] The documentation begins at the time of the initial visit with the examination and evaluation and continues during each visit/encounter through interim notes. Documentation concludes with the discharge summary, or note, following the last encounter in the episode of care (see Chapter 11). Notes written between the initial documentation and discharge note are called interim notes. Interim notes are written in the form of treatment or daily notes, progress notes, regular or formal reassessments, or reevaluations. In order to demonstrate continuity of care being provided and to demonstrate the clinical decision-making process, each interim note refers to and is consistent with the initial documentation and any prior reassessments or reevaluations. Interim notes help tell the patient's "story," and a reader should be able to follow the patient's progress while reading the record. It is also important that each interim note include enough detail to support the skilled interventions provided that day and provide justification for any new, medically necessary interventions added.

TREATMENT AND PROGRESS NOTES

The primary purposes of a treatment or daily note are to document what occurred during a session or encounter in relation to the skilled services provided and to support the billing codes that were used for that particular day. Progress notes, however, are much more extensive and provide more data and detail in all sections, especially the assessment and plan. Progress notes provide changes to the plan of care, address the patient's goals, highlight patient progress, justify the need for continuing skilled care, and show that care is reasonable and necessary. It is important to point out that any information typically required for a progress note may be included in a regular treatment note at any point in the episode of care, but it is not necessary. Although including more detail in treatment notes does help show improvement between the initial documentation and regarding written progress notes. Recall from Chapter 4 that CMS has specific guidelines for treatment notes when treating Medicare beneficiaries in an outpatient setting. Anyone providing services to these individuals should review these guidelines on a regular basis as they do change. Also, anyone providing care to Medicare beneficiaries in other settings should be familiar with the documentation requirements for that setting. For learning note writing, the following rules can be used and then adapted by setting if needed.

Subjective

When writing, the Subjective section of interim notes (treatment of progress notes) includes patient (family member or caregiver) comments that are consistent with and address the chief complaints or issues noted in the initial documentation. Also include patient daily comments and remarks regarding progress, effects of the intervention, functional changes, and status toward his or her goals. Show disablement concepts by detailing how the intervention has brought about changes in patient function, activity limitations, and participation restrictions using the patient's words. Provide, from the patient's perspective, how resolution of impairments is leading to improved function. Finally, include any new complaints, problems, or information relevant to the patient's current condition. Look at the following examples found in the Subjective section of a treatment or progress note.

Comments regarding patient status:

- Patient reported working with his employer regarding return to work. Feeling like he can return to modified duty soon.
- Patient's wife stated she feels that they can manage at home with some assistance from their children.
- Patient reported, "I am feeling stronger."
- Patient reported that she was able to put the dishes into the cabinet last night for the first time since surgery.
- The patient has been a widow for several years and lived alone prior to the accident; however, today reported that her husband is waiting in her room to take her dancing.
- Patient reported that she is able to ambulate more independently in her home and her fear of falling is decreasing.
- The patient's mother reported the patient continues to have problems with wheelchair mobility.

Patient's reaction to interventions provided:

- Patient states that her pain level increased after her last therapy session when a new stretching activity was initiated, but she reports the increase in pain lasted only about an hour and then the pain returned to its normal level.
- Patient reports relief of pain symptoms from 7/10 to 3/10 with the TENS trial following the last visit that allowed her to achieve a full night of sleep.
- The patient reported use of the straight cane has allowed her to be more steady during gait.
- Patient's mother reports the patient is using the involved hand to reach for objects with less cueing.
- Patient stated gait and balance training have helped. States that she can now ambulate without assistance 1000', allowing her to ambulate from the car into her church service independently.
- Patient's husband indicated the leg strengthening exercises have helped in that the patient is now able to transfer in and out of bed without assistance.

New problem(s) or new complaint(s):

- Patient indicated that over the weekend, he noticed increased redness and pain in the lower posterior calf and was diagnosed with a blood clot. States he has not been able to participate in therapy for the last 2 days.
- Patient's mother reported a red spot on the right wrist after wearing the orthosis for 2 hours.
- Patient complains of increased swelling after the addition of the strengthening exercises last session.
- Patient complains of hip pain after initiating the ankle-foot orthosis last visit.

- The nurse reported the patient developed a fever last night and she thinks the incision may be infected.
- The patient's wife reported an increase in difficulty breathing and wheezing following the increased activity in the last session.

Pertinent information not previously documented:

- You are working in an outpatient setting. You have been assisting with the care of a 48-year-old man who injured his back while moving. Today, as you are working with him, he informs you that he had a hernia repair 2 years ago. You know that this information was not included in the initial evaluation or any of the subsequent interim notes. Document: Patient indicated today that he had a hernia repair 2 years ago.
- You have been assisting with the care of an 8-year-old boy in the school system. He has spastic diplegia and a goal is to ambulate between the classroom and cafeteria with supervision and a posterior walker. Today the student tells you that he has started walking with his parents in the evening on a high school track. Document: Today patient reported he has been walking with his parents on a local track.

In most cases, do not use subheadings when writing the Subjective section of interim notes (treatment or progress) but, rather, organize the section by logically grouping together similar information. For example, all information related to the patient's pain (rating, description, and behavior) is grouped together and information related to home environment (distance needed to walk, steps to negotiate, type of flooring) is grouped together. It is advisable, however, to use subheadings to organize information when there are many pieces of subjective data such as in a progress note. Anytime subheadings are included, use those that are consistent with the initial documentation. This will assist the reader in following patient comments throughout the episode of care.

Objective

When writing, the Objective section of interim notes includes (1) results of any screenings, tests, measures, and observations; (2) the patient's functional status; and (3) a clear description of the interventions that are consistent with what is billed on that day of service. In a progress note, the Objective section includes more data and is more thorough than a typical treatment note. When documenting the objective, show consistency by using measures that are consistent with those on the initial and prior documentation. Provide results of any new screenings, tests, and measures when appropriate to show progress (or lack of) toward the established goals.

Document the patient's functional status, including the function, distance or time, type and amount of skilled assistance required, type and amount of cues provided, quality of movement, weight-bearing status, condition under which the function is performed (eg, surfaces), barriers, safety concerns, and any other relevant information to describe the patient's functional status. It is imperative to include the type of assistance provided, especially when you use a unique or complex skill to assist the patient. This helps in showing that skilled assistance was provided. Record functional status especially in areas for which there is an established goal. This allows the reader to see progress made toward goals and that these areas are being addressed during the treatment sessions.

To document interventions, record any information that would allow another therapist to replicate the session. Specific information often includes the following:

[handwritten marginal note: can be used as headings in Rx section]

- The intervention, which falls into one of the following categories[2]:
  - Therapeutic exercise (eg, aerobic or endurance training, balance training, postural training, developmental activities, range of motion, flexibility, motor training, strengthening)
  - Functional training (eg, self-care, home management, work, community, school, play, recreation)
  - Manual therapy techniques (eg, lymphatic draining, manual traction, massage, soft tissue or joint mobilization, passive stretching)
  - Prescription, application, and fabrication of assistive, adaptive, protective, supportive, and prosthetic devices (eg, orthoses, ambulation or transfer aids)
  - Airway clearance techniques (eg, forced expiratory techniques, assisted coughing, drainage, breathing techniques)
  - Integumentary repair and protection techniques (eg, wound care, scar management, debridement of necrotic tissue, dressings)
  - Electrotherapeutic modalities (eg, electrical stimulation, biofeedback, iontophoresis)
  - Physical agents (eg, ultrasound, heat, ice, whirlpool, laser, ultraviolet, compression, standing frames)
- Side and body part (eg, spine, right shoulder, left knee)
- Patient position (eg, prone, side lying) when not performed in the standard position
- Dosage (eg, frequency, intensity, duration, sets, repetitions, settings, parameters)
- Equipment used (eg, weights, assistive or adaptive devices, spirometer, traction device)
- Rest breaks
- A rationale for the intervention if being performed for the first time
- Time for each intervention
- Total treatment time

Use subheadings to clearly differentiate between tests and measures, the patient's functional status, and the interventions provided. When using electronic documentation or standard forms, these sections are divided automatically; however, when writing interim notes by hand or free

typing, clearly differentiate these important aspects of the Objective section.

Document nonprocedural interventions including communication or collaboration with other health care providers or agencies involved in the patient's care, such as personal, phone, or electronic conversations; team meetings; case management; and discharge planning. Document education (patient, family, caregiver, etc) intended to optimize the intervention.[2] Education often relates to the pathology, impairments, activity limitations, participation restrictions, the plan of care, transition to a different role or setting, risk factors, health or wellness needs, precautions, restrictions, safety, and home exercises.[2] Document the specific education that occurred, the type (verbal, handout, brochure, etc), and the patient's (family member's/caregiver's) response to the education. Maintain copies of all written materials provided to patients. Additionally, document the presence of learning barriers.

Assessment

Use the Assessment section of the interim SOAP note to summarize the relevance of data documented within the Subjective and Objective sections. Highlight, or summarize, changes in the patient's status for that day of service (ie, pre- and posttreatment) or since the last visit, the initial session, or last reassessment. These changes include improvements made in impairments, activity limitations, or participation restrictions. When applicable, describe how the physical therapy interventions have helped in bringing about these changes. In the event the patient's status has not changed (ie, plateaued) or has shown a decline in status, use the assessment to describe this plateau or decline and provide a rationale. Like with other sections of the SOAP note, the Assessment section of the progress note is much more extensive and addresses all patient change (or lack thereof) up to that point in the episode of care or since the last progress note. The amount of patient change summarized in a treatment note is an individual therapist decision. For example, a PT may choose to focus on highlighting change in 1 or 2 patient problems in the treatment note but then address all patient problems in the progress note.

When writing the Assessment section of the progress note, summarize the patient's status toward the goals set on the initial documentation. In doing so, indicate if the goal is met, not met (ongoing), or discontinued. Also describe progress made toward established goals. For example, indicate whether the patient is progressing toward goals that have not yet been met. Use the Assessment section of the progress note to justify progress that is faster or slower than what was initially expected, to link ongoing impairment to function, to highlight any new issue(s) interfering with the intervention, and to provide a rationale for discontinuing a goal(s). Use this area to document anything that helps justify ongoing services by giving a very clear picture (in terms others understand) of the patient's progress, ongoing problems and complications, and need for further skilled intervention. Also include the patient's potential for further improvement. Finally, avoid general phrases such as, "The patient tolerated the treatment well."[3] The following examples are typical comments documented in the Assessment section of a treatment note or progress report.

Treatment and progress note examples:

- AROM knee flexion increased 15 degrees after treatment.

- Pain decreased from 6/10 to 2/10 after treatment.

- Gait speed improved 0.2 m/s since yesterday.

- Patient's rate of perceived exertion (RPE) after treatment today was 11; this is improved from yesterday when RPE was 13.

- Patient was able to ambulate to and from the bathroom (~40') with minimal assist and cane today. This is improved from last treatment when he required a standard walker and moderate assist.

Progress note examples:

- Patient has met all established STGs and is progressing toward the LTGs set on the initial documentation.

- Patient has achieved goals 1 to 3. Goals 4 and 5 are ongoing.

- Patient has met goals for transfers and bed mobility. Still needs to work on increasing strength in the lower extremity to prevent the knee from buckling during gait and increase independence in this area.

- Overall, the patient has made good progress toward goals; she is demonstrating a significant reduction in limb volume post-therapy and improved range of motion.

- Patient's progress has been slower than what was originally expected because of transportation issues and unexpected illness that have prevented her from attending regular therapy sessions.

Assessing Change

When assessing the patient for change, one should consider the measurement properties of the various instruments used during the initial examination. Measurement properties that are of particular value when assessing change include "normal" values or scores, degree of error associated with the tests and measures (eg, the standard error of the measurement [SEM]), and the clinical utility, such as the MDC and the instrument's MCID (see Chapter 9). For example, there are normal values associated with range of motion measures, blood pressure, and some patient questionnaires or functional assessments. When assessing and describing a patient's status, document whether a particular measurement falls into the "normal" range. Or, in some cases, you may need to document why a patient's measurements have not returned to the normal value(s).

Familiarity with the degree of error associated with instruments used clinically will also help in assessing change. One common measurement of error found in the literature is the SEM.[4] The SEM is the *amount of error* associated with repeated measurements of the same patient.[4] The value of the SEM gives you the amount of error in the same units as the original test or measure (eg, the SEM for goniometry would be given in degrees).[5,6] There are SEMs associated with single measures as well as with change scores. This is important as you consider the patient's progress. Knowledge of the amount of error associated with a test or measure will help determine whether true change occurred, or if patient change was due merely to error associated with repeated measurements. Let us look at an example from the literature: Authors of a 2006 study published in *Physical Therapy* reported the SEM for measuring gait speed measured on a GaitMat II.[7] The SEM for participant's normal gait speed was 0.04 m/s and 0.05 m/s for faster speeds. We know that any change between baseline and post-intervention speed below the SEM may be indicative of measurement error, rather than true change due to treatment.

Let us apply these results to a patient in a clinical situation:

A patient's gait speed at the initial encounter was 0.82 m/s. After a 4-week physical therapy intervention program, the patient's gait speed was 0.85 m/s, a difference of 0.03 m/s. In this case, yes, the patient has shown a change and a clinician may be inclined to document an improvement in gait speed. However, given the amount of error associated with the measure, the change may be due to measurement error rather than true improvement in speed. Hence, a clinician should not conclude that the patient had made clinically meaningful progress.

After continuing the program for another 2 weeks, the patient's gait speed is reassessed. This time it is 0.92 m/s, a difference of 0.10 m/s since the initial visit. In this case, the clinician could conclude there has been a change outside the margin of error.

Familiarity with the SEM helps clinicians in making decisions with individual patients, allowing him or her to compare the patient's score or change score(s) to the degree of error associated with the test or measure.

In considering patient change, the clinician may also compare the patient's change score with the MDC of the instrument, much like he or she would compare against the SEM. However, the MDC is usually somewhat more conservative than the SEM—meaning, the patient would usually have to change MORE to exceed the MDC than the SEM. Many researchers are investigating the MDC associated with clinical tests and measures. However, this has not always been the case and the MDC is not known for many instruments we use clinically (see Appendix D to see an example of determining the MDC).

Another valuable estimate to help assess clinical change is the MCID. The MCID is used much like the SEM and MDC previously described, in that the patient's change scores are compared to the MCID. Realize, however, that the MCID is an estimate and, like MDC, we do not know the MCID for all tests and measures we use.[7]

More research is needed to determine how values such as SEM, MDC, and MCID can be generalized to patients in a clinical setting. Nevertheless, values identified in the literature provide a starting point for clinicians assessing change using an evidence-based approach. Understanding normal values, the SEM, MDC, and MCID provides us with benchmarks to not only establish goals for a patient but to also summarize meaningful patient change throughout the episode of care.

Plan

In the Plan section of a treatment or progress note, include any new skilled activities or interventions that are planned to address the patient's physical therapy problems. Use the plan to emphasize the progressive nature of the physical therapy services and the episode of care. For example, document the plan to progress the patient to a less supportive assistive device during gait as the patient's balance improves, or document the plan to advance a patient from range of motion to strengthening exercises. Any time new interventions are added or listed in the plan, a justification or explanation provide to show medical necessity. Make modifications to the previous plan of care including any changes to the patient's current intervention(s) or changes in the amount, frequency, or duration of services. In most cases, use the progress note, rather than the treatment note, to make significant changes to the plan of care.

When writing the plan, detailed and specific information is imperative. Clearly state the activities that will occur during upcoming sessions. It is also a good habit to regularly restate the amount, frequency, and duration of physical therapy sessions even if they are unchanged. Generally, avoid frequent use of statements such as, "Continue per plan of care." Repetitive, general entries would require a reviewer to search for the initial documentation in order to locate the current plan, and each note should act as a stand-alone document. The following statements would be appropriate for the Plan section of an interim note:

- Increase weight on terminal knee extensions on the next visit to further increase strengthening.

- Attempt gait with straight cane next session to improve independence.

- Try use of supine stander during the next session to promote weight bearing and upright posture during functional activities.

- Instruct patient's husband in guarding the patient on the stairs in the next session.

- Continue with treatment bid for the next 3 to 5 days at which patient is scheduled for discharge to an inpatient rehabilitation facility.

- Plan to continue with skilled care to instruct the patient and family in safe strengthening and range of motion exercises and to train patient's husband in the use of the Hoyer lift.

Timing Interim Notes

Documentation is required for every patient visit or encounter.[1] The frequency in which progress note are written is dependent on the patient's rate of progress, the frequency of therapy sessions, the setting in which physical therapy is being provided, policies and procedures of the facility, and requirements set forth by regulating agencies and third-party payers. For example, in an outpatient setting, CMS requires a progress note, or report, every 10 treatment sessions.[8] In home health, reassessments and progress reports are also required every 30 days or by the 14th visit. Should services go beyond 14 visits, there must be another reassessment by the 20th visit.[9]

In general, progress notes are written more often when the patient's progress toward the stated goals occurs rapidly. In some situations, each treatment note serves as a progress note. For example, a patient in an acute care setting is recovering from a surgical procedure and significant improvements are seen on a daily basis; therefore, the PT chooses to write a progress note daily to demonstrate this progress. Alternatively, within an inpatient rehabilitation setting, progress notes may be written on a weekly basis in order to report at team conferences, and in a long-term care setting progress notes may be written on a monthly basis. In practice areas that are not bound by policy or regulation to a particular time frame, progress note frequency mirrors the time frame for the established goals but, at minimum, should occur monthly.

REEVALUATIONS

The *Guide to Physical Therapist Practice* defines reexamination as "the process of performing selected test and measures after the initial examination to evaluate progress and to modify or redirect interventions."[2(p47)] Although therapists perform some aspects of reexamination and reevaluation at each patient encounter, there are times when formal reevaluations should occur. Formal reevaluations are required when there has been *any significant change in the patient's status warranting a change in the plan of care.*[8] In addition, reevaluation timing may occur as dictated by state law or facility policy. Recall from Chapter 4 that formal reevaluations are different from regular reassessments. Reevaluations have a separate billing code, whereas regular reassessments are part of the typical episode of care. Even though a reevaluation has a separate billing code, there are stipulations as to whether it will be reimbursed. For example, CMS guidelines indicate that reimbursement for a physical therapy reevaluation requires a significant change in the patient's status that warrants a change in the plan of care (eg, a hospitalization or onset of a new or secondary diagnosis).[8] It is important to be familiar with third-party payer reimbursement guidelines prior to using certain billing codes such as "Physical Therapy Reevaluation."

The documentation of a formal reevaluation includes the same structure and elements described for the initial documentation and for a progress report. The emphasis in a reevaluation, however, is on data that are new or different. The Assessment section clearly describes patient changes that have occurred, goals that have been met, new goals, adaptations to the plan of care (goals, interventions, frequency or duration of care), and the patient's continued need for skilled services. All changes to the plan of care are justified by evidence provided within the Subjective and Objective sections of the note.

LETTERS

As a PT, you may find yourself writing letters to various individuals involved in the health care of the patient/client. In any setting, as a professional courtesy, you will write letters to physicians of patients you are treating to provide a status update. This can happen at the onset of physical therapy services following the initial examination, intermittently throughout the episode of care, and/or at discharge. It is also beneficial for the PT to communicate to a patient's physician regarding physical therapy interventions provided even if the patient has sought physical therapy via direct access. Communicating in this way helps to build mutual respect between health care providers and, in turn, helps to facilitate the patient's overall health care.

When writing a letter to a physician, clearly and concisely tailor the information to address the areas in which the physician is most likely concerned or interested. Include a brief introduction and statement giving the patient information. Provide relevant subjective comments, objective findings, present problems, your overall impression, and your plan. Finally, as a courtesy, thank the physician for the referral (Example 10-1). Occasionally, PTs will create form letters and templates to facilitate the letter-writing process, and electronic documentation software often includes standard letters and forms to physicians that are populated with data from a previous progress or treatment note. Case managers and third-party payers may also request similar letters. Information provided in these types of letters is tailored to address the questions and concerns of the individual requesting the information. Keep a copy of any such written communication in the patient's physical therapy record.

SUMMARY

Interim notes include (1) treatment or daily notes that serve as a record of care provided and billed for that day of service using skilled terminology, (2) progress notes that justify ongoing services, and (3) reevaluations are done after a change in patient status. Interim documentation may also include letters and communication notes to other individuals involved with the patient when needed.

For treatment or daily notes, the clinician providing the intervention—whether that is the PT or the PTA—completes the documentation. If more than one therapist treats a patient in a single session, PT or PTA, then both individuals should authenticate, or sign, the documentation. Within this interim documentation, the PT is solely responsible for modifying the plan of care, interpreting new orders, performing regular reassessments and formal reevaluations, and writing the Assessment and Plan sections of the progress notes. A PTA can write treatment notes and, where allowed by law, the PTA may write the Assessment and Plan sections of a treatment note. Within this documentation, a PTA can document a need for changes to the plan of care, but it is the sole responsibility of the PT to follow-up with the reassessment and record changes to the plan of care. In some cases, a PT may use a PTA to assist with data collection and documentation in the Subjective and Objective sections of the progress note, but the Assessment and Plan are the responsibility of the PT.

Interim notes are written in a manner to show consistency with the initial documentation so as to tell a story of the patient's episode of care. Interim notes reflect disablement concepts, clinical problem solving, and skilled care provided. Each note serves as evidence that will ultimately justify the patient's care.

Example 10-1. Sample Letter to a Physician

Dear Dr. Smith,

I am writing to provide an update on your patient Richard Jones (DOB: 3/3/1936), whom you referred to physical therapy for treatment following a right ankle fracture.

At this time (8 weeks post-fracture) he reports pain as 3/10 and notes improved function in the home and community. He has resumed independent ADL and some home tasks. His AROM for DF is 10 degrees, PF is 50 degrees, inversion is 20 degrees, and eversion is 5 degrees. Strength is 4/5 throughout, and he is able to ambulate full weight bearing without an assistive device. His balance is fair and he is independent with all mobility on level surfaces.

He continues to have difficulty on uneven surfaces including ambulation on uneven ground. This is a problem since he works as a farmer. I would like to continue treatment 1-2 times weekly to progress strength, proprioception, higher level balance activities, and ankle strategies to improve ambulation on all surfaces.

Please contact me at 304-667-1717 if you have any questions or want to discuss this patient further. Thank you for this referral and I look forward to continuing to work with him.

Respectfully,

Sue Smith, PT

REVIEW QUESTIONS

1. List the different types of interim notes. What is the purpose of each?

   daily notes, re-evaluation, progress note (re-assessment)

2. Compare and contrast a treatment note and a progress note. In your discussion, include the purpose of each and the contents of each.

3. Is a summary of patient progress a requirement for a treatment note or progress note? Who decides the amount of progress summarized in a treatment note?

4. What information should be included in the Objective section of a treatment or progress note?

   results of tests & measures, pt's functional status, interventions for DOS

5. In what type of note are the patient's goals addressed and updated?

   progress notes

6. What information is required for documenting an intervention?

   any info that would allow another therapist to replicate it

7. When and where should the justification for integrating a new intervention be provided in the documentation?

8. Compare and contrast the roles of the PT and PTA regarding interim documentation.

9. How is a reevaluation different from a regular reassessment?

10. Of the following, which can be billed to the patient using a separate billing code: ongoing weekly assessment, a formal reassessment, and/or a formal reevaluation?

APPLICATION EXERCISES

1. Write the following information in a more clear, concise manner, as it would appear in the medical record. Replace the percentage of assistance provided with min, mod, or max assist where appropriate.

   a. You are working with a patient in an outpatient clinic with a diagnosis of right bicipital tendonitis. She tells you that she has been working on the home exercises and overall her arm is feeling much better. She reports improvements in dressing and fixing her hair. She reports her current pain to be 3/10 on a verbal pain scale. She says that she has trouble reaching into overhead cabinets and shelves. Her treatment consisted of phonophoresis over the anterior shoulder for 8 minutes, 50% duty cycle with the intensity set at 1.5 w/cm². This was followed by active scapular retraction and protraction, prone horizontal abduction, and external rotation with yellow exercise band for 2 sets of 10 repetitions with verbal and tactile cues for positioning. She also received manual therapy including grades 2 and 3 anteroposterior and inferior joint mobilizations to improve joint movement and decrease pain. The total exercise session lasted 30 minutes. The treatment concluded with ice for 15 minutes.

   b. You are working with an inpatient with Guillain-Barré syndrome. He reports that he is doing better today with much less fatigue after the session yesterday. His therapeutic exercise consisted of ankle pumps, active hip abduction, heel slides, bridging, and knee extension at the edge of the mat (3 sets of 10 repetitions). After the exercises, you worked on functional training including transfers from the bed to and from the wheelchair using a stand pivot transfer. The patient required ~25% to 30% assistance from 1 therapist, although you did have to block his knees because of quadriceps weakness. At the end of the session, the patient required 50% to 60% assist to transfer back to bed because of mild fatigue. He positioned himself in bed with verbal cues and use of the side rails for assist to scoot. His ability to transfer has not improved in the last week. The plan is to work on gait training in the afternoon session.

c. You are working with an elderly woman in the acute care setting who has suffered a right CVA 3 days ago. The patient is cooperative and complains of lack of mobility and function. You perform passive and active assistive range of motion on her left upper and lower extremities using facilitation techniques to promote active movement. The patient was not showing signs of abnormal tone or reflex development. You performed 30 repetitions for the upper and lower extremities. You also provided manual resistance for the right upper and lower extremities for 30 repetitions. You provided stretching to the left heel cords to increase joint range of motion to allow normal stance. The stretch was performed 5 times, holding for 30 seconds each time. The patient transferred out of bed with minimal assist of 1 to the wheelchair with stabilization for her left knee and trunk support. She ambulated twice in the parallel bars 8 feet with right upper extremity support. She required minimal assist of 1 for trunk support and moderate assist of 1 at the left lower extremity for swing, placement of the foot, and knee stabilization. The plan is for discharge in the next 1 to 2 days to inpatient rehabilitation. Your more immediate plan is to work with her twice daily on range of motion and mobility skills until discharge.

d. You are working with a patient 3 days status post–right total knee replacement in the therapy gym. Pain rating is 6/10. States she has rheumatoid arthritis (RA) and has difficulty getting moving. She states she wants to be discharged to home to live alone. She has noticeable swelling and limited range of motion in the knee and ankle. Active range of motion in the right knee measure 5 to 65 degrees. She transfers wheelchair to and from the mat with you providing 25% assistance because of her left lower extremity weakness and difficulty standing. She transferred sit to and from supine with you performing 50% assistance because of her inability to lift the right leg onto the mat table. She performed 2 sets of 10 repetitions of the total knee exercises and ambulated

50 feet, twice with a standard walker, putting only 50% of her body weight on the involved extremity. She required assistance for sequencing the walker and her steps to allow unweighting the involved extremity. She received ice for 15 minutes to her knee. You suspect her limited mobility and the fact that she lives alone will require her to remain an inpatient longer than normal. You also suspect the RA may be limiting her progress. You will plan to continue with increasing ROM and independence with mobility until d/c and recommend a short-term post-acute care placement until independence improves.

e. You are working with a patient recently hospitalized for pneumonia, mild congestive heart failure and dementia, and lower extremity weakness. She tells you that she is looking forward to going home where she lives alone. She complains of some difficulty breathing during the session. She is using oxygen provided by a nasal cannula on 2 L. The patient walked 150' where she required contact guard assist and monitoring because of her shortness of breath. You are monitoring her respiratory rate (14 breaths/min prior to ambulation and 20 after). You also monitored her oxygen saturation level (94% prior to treatment and 90% after). She also demonstrated swaying during gait and complains of dizziness when turning her head during ambulation. You feel that she is not ready to go home alone and should have continued therapy after discharge because of balance and endurance issues. Your plan is to continue working on increasing endurance and balance twice daily and to work with case management on transfer to the hospital's skilled unit.

2. Using the initial documentation on pp. 38 and 39 (Chapter 4, Amputation) to make comparisons, rewrite the following information into a progress report.

a. The patient is now 2 weeks s/p right transtibial amputation and is still in the inpatient rehabilitation setting. He is continuing to complain of phantom pain (he rates at 4/10) and sensation from the right foot. It resolves if he "squeezes" his residual limb. You are planning to attend a team conference for him on the following day, so you decide to take some objective measurements. Right active range of motion is hip flexion 120 degrees, extension 5 degrees, abduction 40 degrees, adduction 10 degrees, knee flexion 130 degrees, knee extension −5 degrees. Passive range of motion is right knee extension 0 degrees. Strength in the right lower extremity for hip flexion is 4/5; for extension he holds against moderate resistance in side-lying position, for abduction he holds against moderate resistance in the side-lying position, for knee extension he holds against minimal resistance in seated position, and for knee flexion he holds against moderate resistance in the side-lying position. The patient cannot lay prone because of pulmonary problems and difficulty breathing when in this position. The incision is healing well. There is no drainage and no signs or symptoms of infection. It is moderately adhered to the underlying tissue and hypersensitive to pressure. Residual limb girth is 40 cm at the right knee joint, 41 cm 2" below, and 42 cm 4" below. The patient can move and transfer in and out of bed independently to a bedside commode or chair. He can manage the wheelchair parts with verbal cueing. He propels the wheelchair 50' independently on level surfaces and carpet and then requires a rest. He can ambulate 75' with a standard walker with supervision × 1 and his balance is good. Assist is required because he fatigues quickly and needs cueing for sequencing the walker. Gait training lasted 15' and other functional training lasted 20'. You spent the next 15 minutes on patient education and exercise. The patient is independent with residual limb care and using the shrinker sock. You have also made initial contact with a prosthetist regarding this patient. He is planning on going home in 1 to 2 weeks. The total session lasted 60 minutes. You also plan to continue with skilled intervention for safely progressing exercises and endurance to improve mobility and independence in the home and to work on pain and edema control to prepare limb for prosthesis and increase standing and mobility activities.

b. The patient is now 10 weeks s/p right transtibial amputation and is being seen as an outpatient. He has been receiving treatment as an outpatient for the last 2 weeks when he received his prosthesis. His goals for the outpatient setting (to be met over the next 2 months) are as follows:

i. Normal range of motion in the residual limb to allow independence with prosthesis and a normal, efficient gait pattern.

ii. Strength of the right lower extremity will be 5/5 to promote independence with prosthesis and a normal, efficient gait pattern.

iii. Tolerate 8 hours of continuous prosthetic use without skin breakdown.

iv. The patient will demonstrate good balance as evidenced by a score <14 seconds on the Timed Up and Go (TUG).

v. Ambulate >300 m on the 6-minute walk test.

vi. Score >35 on the Amputee Mobility Predictor (AMP).

c. Use the following information to write a progress note for this patient. Assume you have been treating this patient since his inpatient stay. Use the data in Application Exercise 2a as a comparison. Convert strength descriptions to manual muscle test grades. Include STGs. The patient is continuing to complain of phantom pain and sensation from the right foot occasionally, but it has decreased to 2/10. He is reporting improvements in his home environment including ambulation with the crutches for short distances and ability to wear the prosthesis for 2 to 3 hours. Reports his grandson has been staying with him to provide assist and transportation to therapy. Right active range of motion is hip flexion 120 degrees, extension 10 degrees, abduction 40 degrees, adduction 10 degrees, knee flexion 140 degrees, knee extension 0 degrees. Strength in the right LE hip flexion 4/5; extension holds against moderate resistance in side-lying position; abduction holds against moderate resistance in side-lying position; knee extension holds against moderate resistance in seated position; knee flexion holds against maximum resistance in side-lying position. The incision is not adhered to the underlying tissue and sensitivity has subsided. Residual limb girth is 40 cm at the knee joint, 39 cm 2" below, and 39 cm 4" below. He is independent with all wheelchair parts and transfer. He propels the wheelchair 500' independently on level surfaces and carpet. He can ambulate 150' with axillary crutches with supervision × 1 and good balance without the prosthesis. You spent the next 30 minutes on prosthetic training. He requires minimal assist to don and doff the socket and secure the supracondylar cuff suspension. He ambulates 50' with the prosthesis on and with axillary crutches with minimal assist for advancing the prosthesis. He is ambulating with an abducted gait on the prosthetic side. His TUG Score is 22 seconds. His AMP score is 32. You would like to begin stair training with the prosthesis and advancing his gait skills (curbs, ramps, etc). You would like to see him twice weekly. His motivation is good and you believe his potential to improve is good. You spend 10 minutes educating the patient on skin precautions after removing the prosthesis and 15 minutes on exercises where he requires facilitation and manual cueing for proper performance. Minimal detectable change for outcome measures in this population are 45 m for the 6-minute walk test, 3.6 seconds for the TUG, and 3.4 for the AMP.[10]

3. Use the initial documentation you created in Chapter 9 Application Exercise #6 (CVA) and create a progress note based on the following information. On the third day of treatment, the patient states he feels he is getting stronger and is looking forward to continuing his recovery. The patient and his wife stated they discussed inpatient rehabilitation placement with case manager. The patient's wife states

she is concerned about how they will manage in the long run. She says that their son and daughter-in-law are able to provide some assistance but she will be the primary caregiver. In therapy today you worked on his bed mobility and transfers for 15 minutes. You worked on gait for 15'. He needed moderate assistance when scooting up and down and side to side in bed. He was able to roll to the right without any assistance and was safe with the activity. He required minimal assistance when rolling to the left. The patient still displays significant edema (girth 43.6 cm) in his right hand and forearm and reports that he forgets to use his positioning devices in bed and in the wheelchair. He required minimal assistance to transfer supine to sit. He requires minimal assistance when performing a sit to stand transfer and moderate assistance with a stand pivot transfer from the therapy mat into the wheelchair. He ambulated with a quad cane with min (a) × 1 to support his trunk and assist with balance and mod (a) × 1 to advance and stabilize the right leg. He ambulated 20' × 2 and then required a rest break. He requires a rest break 4× in a 30-minute session. You tell him you will see him again in the afternoon to work on more therapeutic exercises and to ambulate. You educated the patient's wife regarding his need for supervision and constant verbal cues because he is impulsive and unsafe at times.

REFERENCES

1. American Physical Therapy Association. Guidelines: Physical Therapy Documentation of Patient/Client Management BOD G03-05-16-41. http://www.apta.org/uploadedFiles/APTAorg/About_Us/Policies/BOD/Practice/DocumentationPatientClientMgmt.pdf. Accessed May 16, 2012.

2. American Physical Therapy Association. *Guide to Physical Therapist Practice.* 2nd ed. Alexandria, VA: APTA; 2003.

3. Clifton DW. "Tolerated treatment well" may no longer be tolerated. *PT Magazine.* 1995;3(10):24.

4. MacDermid JC, Stratford P. Applying evidence on outcome measures to hand therapy practice. *J Hand Ther.* 2004;17:165-173.

5. Finch E, Brooks D, Stratford PW, Mayo NE. *Physical Rehabilitation Outcomes Measures.* 2nd ed. Philadelphia, PA: Lippincott Williams & Wilkins; 2002.

6. Domholdt E. *Physical Therapy Research: Principles and Applications.* 2nd ed. Philadelphia, PA: W.B. Saunders; 2000.

7. Palombaro KM, Craik RL, Mangione KK, Tomlinson JD. Determining meaningful changes in gait speed after hip fracture. *Phys Ther.* 2006;86:809-816.

8. Centers for Medicare & Medicaid Services. Covered medical and other health services. *Medicare Benefit Policy Manual.* Publication 100-02. http://www.cms.gov/Regulations-and-Guidance/Guidance/Manuals/Downloads/bp102c15.pdf. Accessed May 16, 2012.

9. Centers for Medicare & Medicaid Services. Home health services. *Medicare Benefit Policy Manual.* Publication 100-02. http://www.cms.gov/Regulations-and-Guidance/Guidance/Manuals/Downloads/bp102c07.pdf. Accessed May 16, 2012.

10. Reference: Resnik L, Borgia M. Reliability and outcome measures for people with lower-limb amputations: distinguishing true change from statistical error. *Phys Ther.* 2011;91:555-565.

Chapter 11

Patient Outcomes and Discharge Summaries

Mia L. Erickson, PT, EdD, CHT, ATC

CHAPTER OUTLINE

CHAPTER OBJECTIVES

Upon completion of this chapter, the reader will be able to:
1. Define outcome.
2. Recognize the importance of examining outcomes for cohorts and individual patients.
3. Describe the benefits of using functional assessments as outcomes measures.
4. Construct an appropriate discharge summary.
5. Integrate measures of clinical change such as MDC and MCID in outcomes.
6. Realize the use of functional assessments in quality initiatives.
7. Describe the barriers associated with using functional assessments in outcomes data collection.
8. Outline practical suggestions for establishing a clinical outcomes data collection process.

Erickson ML, Utzman RR, McKnight R. *Physical Therapy Documentation:*
From Examination to Outcome, Second Edition (pp 117-124).
© 2014 SLACK Incorporated.

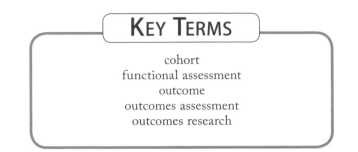

KEY TERMS

cohort
functional assessment
outcome
outcomes assessment
outcomes research

Over the last decades, outcomes assessment and outcomes research have become mainstays in physical therapy practice, research, and policy making. A patient's outcome is the end result of his or her health care for a given injury, disease, or condition. The *Guide to Physical Therapist Practice* defines outcome as the "impact," or end result, of patient/client management.[1] There are many different ways to assess a patient's outcome. Physical therapists are often interested in examining the effects of the intervention we provide, whether it is a procedural intervention, such as therapeutic exercise or a specific modality, or nonprocedural intervention, such as patient education. There are many ways to examine the effects of our intervention. At the conclusion of the episode of care, we may look at a variety of factors, or outcome variables, such as the patient's pathology, impairments, functional status, risk reduction, overall health or wellness, or satisfaction, to name a few.[1] Additional outcome variables important to PTs as well as others involved in the patient's care include quality and value of health care provided,[2] especially with regard to overall cost of the intervention(s) and degree of improvement attained. Other outcome variables include things such as time lost from work, lost wages, return-to-work status, number of visits or sessions, hospital readmission, or total cost of treatment provided. When examining the effects of the intervention, it is important to remember that the outcome is determined by patient factors, behavior, or status and not by provider behavior. For example, a PT measuring outcomes attempts to determine effectiveness of an intervention so he measures the patient's functional performance, impairments, return to independent living, and societal integration following a traumatic injury. Measurements of provider actions, such as whether the PT is tracking patient education, are not patient outcomes indicators.[3]

A patient determines the effects of treatment based on things that he or she cares most about such as functional change and improved quality of life.[2] In the late 1980s, medical professionals, including rehabilitation professionals, began using functional assessment as a means for measuring outcome in order to capture things that matter most to patients.[2,4] Functional measures consider the patient's perspective of his or her abilities and overall well-being and they provide a powerful assessment of patient change during the time the treatment was provided.[5] Functional assessments also help health care providers communicate the patient's functional status with others. In using functional terminology we provide insight, with a better description of how the injury or illness affects the patient's

day-to-day life, in terms lay people understand.[6] Without functional measures "payers cannot understand us when we attempt to communicate."[5(p1)] The aforementioned benefits of functional assessment, however, are not intended to say that impairment measures are not important. In fact, one should integrate both together as they are relevant to research, practice, and development of the profession's scientific body of knowledge.[6]

DOCUMENTING OUTCOMES

PTs examine outcomes for cohorts or individual patients.[3,7] A cohort is a group of patients with a similar injury, diagnosis, or characteristics (eg, rotator cuff repair, traumatic brain injury). One way to assess outcomes for a cohort is to perform the same tests and measures on each group member at the same point in time. For example, a therapist examining the effectiveness of a balance and falls program might assess participant's fall risk prior to participation and again 4, 8, and 12 weeks after beginning participation. Additionally, one could perform the same measures at some point following program completion, such as 1 year after completing the program. Clinicians and researchers employ measures in this manner to provide insight to program and treatment effectiveness. Data are used in program quality improvement, marketing materials, publications, and professional presentations.

Individual patient outcomes are considered throughout the episode of care. First, the therapist considers "an expected outcome" for every patient that is articulated through outcome, or discharge, goals. At each reassessment, the PT considers and documents progress toward the outcome goals by comparing current and prior subjective and objective data. At the end of the episode of care, the PT documents the patient's outcome, or end result, in a discharge summary. The following section describes components of a properly constructed discharge summary, and a documentation template for creating a discharge summary can be found in Table 11-1.

The Discharge Summary

Subjective

The discharge summary includes the final subjective remarks given in a manner similar to the initial documentation. It includes comments that will allow direct

	Table 11-1 **Discharge Summary Template**	
Subjective	Provide patient/family/caregiver remarks regarding final status, improvement, independence, etc
	Provide information regarding the benefits of treatment, improved daily living, performance of functional tasks
	Provide status regarding chief complaints and functional problems identified in the initial documentation
	Provide any other subjective information that gives insight to the patient's final status
Objective	Document results of relevant tests and measures that are consistent with initial, or prior, documentation
	Document intervention(s) provided on the final day of service including patient-related instruction
	Summarize the intervention provided throughout the episode of care
Assessment	Give the reason for discharge
	Summarize the effects of the intervention on impairment, function, risks, health and wellness, societal resources, or any other aims of the intervention
	Summarize patient change using measures from the literature (ie, normal values, minimal detectable change, clinically important difference)
	Give the status toward the discharge or outcome goals set by the PT
	Describe any remaining issues, problems, or goals that have not been met and provide a rationale
	Describe any comorbidity or factor(s) complicating the episode of care
Plan	List any patient, provider, family member, or caregiver activity that will take place following the final session
	Give the discharge destination (eg, inpatient rehabilitation) or participation status (eg, return to work)

comparisons between the initial or prior documentation and the final documentation in the areas of patient complaints, concerns, and goals. It includes patient or family members' remarks regarding the patient's overall improvement, the current functional status, and any changes brought on by the intervention(s). The discharge summary also provides comments given by the patient, family, or caregiver describing functional improvements brought on by the reduction of impairments. Look at the following examples.

Example 11-1. Discharge Subjective

- Patient reports he is now able to get in and out of bed independently and no longer requires assist from wife.
- Patient reports that all rehabilitation goals met.
- Patient states that stretching brought on improved knee range of motion and allows improvement in ascending and descending stairs.

- Patient's daughter indicated that family training helped her in increasing safety during transferring the patient and that she can do it without difficulty.
- Patient stated that balance training has helped her to feel more "steady" and she reports a decrease in the amount of "stumbling" over the last 3 months.

Objective

In addition to the final subjective status, the discharge documentation includes results of objective tests and measures used to make comparisons between initial, prior, and current impairments and functional status. It includes new tests and measures when needed, such as strength or muscle testing, that were not appropriate at the initial visit because of surgical precautions. All tests and measures accurately reflect the patient's status at the conclusion of the episode of care. In the Objective section of the discharge summary, the PT summarizes the skilled care provided throughout the episode to give a final justification for why it was medically necessary. This is not an "all inclusive" list but a summary describing important components of care provided. The final documentation also includes a list of skilled treatment provided and billed on the final day of service. Subheadings or section headers are used to differentiate between services provided during the final encounter and those provided in other sessions.

Example 11-2. Interventions Documented at Discharge

Today's treatment: 15 min of therapeutic activities on the mat working on lower extremity strength to facilitate the quads, gluts, and hip abductors; also included and sit to stand transfers to increase performance and strength. Patient was instructed in and performed final home exercises without difficulty (attached handout) for 15 min. Patient's daughter was instructed in car transfers and methods to safely assist the patient for 15 min. Total time today 45 min.

Summary of episode of care: Patient's episode of care has included various activities to improve strength of the lower extremities to improve mobility in/out of bed and during ambulation; balance training to decrease her fall risk; and functional training to facilitate independent living.

However, there may be times when a final reassessment is not performed, such as when the patient is discharged by the physician or the patient stops coming to therapy. In these cases, the PT incorporates data from the previous measurements and provides the date it was recorded.

Example 11-3. No Discharge Reassessment

The patient did not return for her final visit, objective measurements show status at the time of the last visit, 1 week ago.

Patient discharged from unit suddenly and formal discharge assessment was not performed. Objective measures are from last session, 5/15/12.

Assessment

The PT documents the Assessment and Plan sections of the discharge summary. In the Assessment section, he or she provides a reason for the patient's discharge and a summary of meaningful patient change that occurred as a result of the episode of care. There are many reasons why patients are discharged from physical therapy services. Those include, but are not limited to, all established goals were met, the patient or family/caregiver declined further intervention, or the patient became unable to participate. In this section, the PT summarizes specific changes occurring in the patient's initial pathology, impairments, function, risk, overall health or wellness, or societal resources (eg, assistance needed) since the onset of treatment (Table 11-2).[1] The PT uses his or her knowledge of the scientific evidence to determine whether clinically significant, meaningful changes occurred and describes data using the evidence if appropriate. This aids in describing the effects of the intervention on impairment reduction and functional improvement. Also, the PT provides the patient's status toward the outcome goals (eg, goal met, goal ongoing, progress made, goal discontinued) and overall satisfaction with the improvement. In addition, the final documentation includes any remaining issues, problems, or goals that have not been achieved and the reason(s), such as a comorbidity or complication.

Example 11-4. Discharge Assessment 1

The patient has met all goals for physical therapy except for return to work; however, his case manager is working on a placement for him to begin right away. The interventions have helped in increasing mobility, strength, and functional restoration. His wrist mobility is now WNL. He also demonstrated a significant improvement (> 50#) in grip strength and it is now 80% of his opposite side. His functional assessment decreased from 85% to 5% suggesting minimal to no disability. He is also independent with his home program.

Example 11-5. Discharge Assessment 2

The patient has met all goals established and has demonstrated significant improvement since the initial visit. Following exercises and functional training, she now demonstrates the ability to move in and out of bed independently, ambulates household distances independently and safely with a standard walker, and ascends and descend stairs with minimal supervision provided by her husband. She performs all exercises independently without cueing. Today her husband demonstrated independence with the car transfer and all questions were answered. Patient will still need to work on her goal of independent community ambulation.

Table 11-2

Domains Addressed During Physical Therapy Interventions and Sample Documentation of the Patient's Status at Discharge

If your intervention addresses . . .	Sample Documentation
Pathology	• Patient no longer showing signs or symptoms of complex regional pain syndrome
	• Patient no longer showing signs or symptoms of patellar tendinitis
Impairment	• Range of motion of the (L) shoulder is WNL in all planes and equal to the (R)
	• Strength (L) elbow is 5/5 in all directions
Activity limitation	• Patient can ascend and descend stairs independently
	• Patient can perform all transfers without limitation
Participation restriction	• Patient now able to participate in all school-related activities without limitation
	• Patient now safe with unlimited community ambulation
Risk reduction and prevention	• Patient now independent with all lifting tasks and shows good body mechanics
Health, wellness, and fitness	• Patient is independent with fitness program
Societal resources	• Patient is independent in use of public transportation
Patient satisfaction	• Patient is pleased with her status and feels that she can discontinue therapy

Plan

In the Plan section of the discharge documentation, the PT provides a list of anything that will take place following the final session with the patient. Depending on the patient, the length and contents of this section will vary. Examples of information include any plans for intervention at another setting (eg, inpatient rehabilitation, home health care, outpatient therapy); independent or maintenance intervention through a home program; obtaining assistive or adaptive equipment; and transition into participation such as returning to work, school, recreation, or community activities. The PT documents any plans for working toward goals that have not been met, referring the patient to another provider or individual who will assist the patient, and communicating with other individuals regarding the patient's care or status.

Example 11-6. Plan from Discharge Note 1

Patient will be discharged from physical therapy to an independent home exercise program and will return to work at his prior level of employment. He will call if questions arise.

Example 11-7. Plan from Discharge Note 2

Patient will continue with therapy services through outpatient day program here at the hospital. He will receive further intervention for planning for community integration such as identifying appropriate employment. Will speak with case manager about physical capabilities to assist with this transition.

OUTCOMES AND HEALTH CARE ADMINISTRATION

Clinicians, managers, and payers alike are interested in patients' outcome data from an administrative perspective. For example, functional measures have become associated with measuring health care quality and provider performance.[8] Administrators use data to assess clinic-wide or individual provider credibility and accountability, inform decision making about specific interventions or programs, and improve program quality. Additionally, CMS is including functional assessments as a quality indicator in the Physician Quality Reporting System program.[9,10]

There are considerations, however, with using functional assessments to assess quality. First, clinicians should implement measures and instruments repeatedly, so quality assessment is based on the patient's change over time rather than on a single evaluation.[11] Also, one must realize that longer periods of observation minimize the connection between the outcome(s) and the care provided. Extraneous factors affecting both patients and providers begin weighing more heavily as time goes on, making it more difficult to draw conclusions about the quality of providers and care rendered.[11] Patient factors such as disease progression, comorbidities, co-interventions, adherence, motivation, socioeconomic status, educational level, and payer source may affect outcomes data either positively or negatively. Provider and organizational factors such as documentation procedures, measurement variability between providers, differing intervention strategies, time allotment, data storage, and types of measurements selected to determine outcome also influence data. In addition, "from both a conceptual and methodological perspective, outcomes assessment must take into account all of the services received from all providers involved in the patient care process."[12(pp111-112)] This is important in multidisciplinary settings such as inpatient rehabilitation, where a patient may be receiving multiple services such as physical therapy, occupational therapy, speech therapy, neuropsychology, nutritional services, and others. Clinicians must consider these issues since "collecting and reporting bad data simply because it is available does nothing to aid in informed decision making or maximization of outcome effect."[5(p302)]

A PLAN FOR ASSESSING OUTCOMES

Prior to establishing an outcomes measurement plan, determine (1) its purpose, (2) the source of data, (3) the procedures and/or individual(s) responsible for data collection, and (4) the individual(s) responsible for storing and analyzing data. Address both practical and logistical factors by asking who, what, where, when, why, and how. For example[11]:

1. Who will collect the data?

   Examples: PT during the initial visit, office staff during initial paperwork

2. What kind of data/measurements will be collected?

   Examples: Impairments, function, self-report questionnaires, global health-related quality of life questionnaires, disease-specific questionnaires

3. Are measurements reliable and valid? What is the associated error, MDC, or MCID?

4. What are the hallmarks of a "good" or "bad" outcome?

5. Where will data be collected?

   Examples: Clinic or hospital, paper or electronic, completion at home

6. When will data be collected?

   Examples: Initial visit, 4 weeks, after x number of visits

7. Why will you collect data?

   Examples: How will the data be used? What is the purpose? To whom will data be provided?

8. How will data be collected?

   Examples: Procedures for ongoing data collection, tracking when data need to be collected

Regardless of benefits that arise from good data collection and reporting, barriers exist.[3] Barriers include personnel resistance to implementing new data collection procedures; time needed for performing, documenting, storing, retrieving, analyzing, and reporting data; and the need for consistency in patient coding (ie, ICD-9) to facilitate data retrieval. In addition, there may be direct and indirect costs associated with new equipment, instruments, personnel, or training. Another consideration is whether to use a computerized outcomes management software package. These can be expensive because of associated costs of hardware, software, upgrades, and report generation.

SUMMARY

Functional assessment as a means of outcomes data collection is becoming more widespread, and the use of patient questionnaires and performance measures is growing. Whether data are collected for groups or individual patients, in implementing these measures a clinician needs to identify valid instruments reflecting the aspects of health he or she is interested in measuring, as well as their associated measurement properties. These can be used to establish goals or benchmarks as well as to describe meaningful patient change. There are many uses for outcomes data and clinicians need to consider the entire process when implementing.

APPLICATION EXERCISES

1. Identify one functional outcome test or measure for each of the following settings. Research its measurement properties. Give the following measurement properties: SEM, MDC, and MCID. Determine if it is generic or disease (body-part) specific. Determine the administration technique (ie, patient performance or self-report).

   a. Acute care setting
   b. Inpatient rehabilitation unit
      i.   Neurological disorder
      ii. Musculoskeletal disorder
   c. Skilled nursing unit

REVIEW QUESTIONS

1. In your own words, define outcome.

2. What are the benefits of assessing patient function?

3. List the components of a discharge summary.
   Subjective, objective, assessment, plan

4. How are disablement concepts integrated into a discharge summary?
   in the assessment of the note

5. Why is consistency between the initial, subsequent (or interim), and discharge documentation important?
   to better evaluate outcomes

6. Give 3 different patient cohorts. Provide examples of medical record data that would be useful in examining treatment effectiveness for these groups.

7. What is the importance of knowing the standard error of the measurement (SEM) when assessing a patient's outcome?

8. How can the MDC and MCID be used in assessing outcome?

9. How can outcomes assessments be used in quality initiatives?

10. Describe some barriers associated with outcomes data collection.

    d. Home health
    e. Outpatient adult ambulatory clinic
      i. Upper extremity
      ii. Lower extremity
      iii. Spine
      iv. General
    f. Cardiopulmonary patient (Dx: COPD) in home health
    g. Pediatric outpatient clinic—neurological disorders
    h. Pediatric outpatient clinic—musculoskeletal disorders
    i. Pediatric school setting—ages 5 to 9 years old
    j. Early intervention (birth to 3 years old)

2. Identify a setting (like one listed in question 1) and a common diagnosis seen in that particular setting. Determine how you could go about implementing an outcomes assessment program for those patients.

3. Identify one clinician in your area and interview him or her regarding the use of outcomes assessment tools in the clinical setting. What instruments does he or she use? How are they used (ie, when is it administered, who administers it, how is it stored, etc)? How has it influenced his or her practice? How has it influenced reimbursement? How is it incorporated into his or her documentation?

4. Using the initial documentation from Chapter 9, complete a discharge summary using the information here.

One week later after the initial examination, the patient is being discharged to inpatient rehabilitation. You work with him just prior to his discharge. He states that he has made a lot of recovery in 1 week. During the discharge examination you identify the following. He continues to have pitting edema in the (R) hand and forearm and tends to keep his (R) UE in a dependent position. He maintains the extremity in the appropriate position with verbal cueing. The figure 8 hand girth is (R) 53.5 cm. His sensation is diminished to light touch, deep pressure localization, proprioception, and kinesthesia through the (R) UE and LE. Muscle tone shows grade of 0 on the upper extremities and 1 on the lower extremities using the Modified Ashworth Scale. At the (R) shoulder there is a 1 finger width sulcus at the GH joint. Muscle strength in the shoulder, elbow, and wrist remain 2–/5 and finger flexion is 1/5. Hip strength is 3/5 for flexion and extension and 3–/5 for abduction, adduction, internal rotation, and external rotation. Knee flexion is 3–/5 and extension is 3–/5. Ankle strength is 2–/5 for dorsiflexion and plantarflexion. He is able to stand without physical assistance or UE support at a quad cane with supervision with erect posture. During his therapy session today, the patient required minimal assistance of 1 with scooting up, down, and side-to-side. He was independent with rolling to the right and required minimal assist of 1 to roll to the left and for supine to sit transfers. He requires supervision when performing a sit-to-stand transfer and stand pivot transfer from the bed into the wheelchair for safety. He ambulated with a quad cane with min (a) × 1 to support his trunk and assist with balance and min (a) × 1 to advance and stabilize the right leg. He ambulated 35' × 2 and then required a rest break. He requires 2 rest breaks in a 30-minute session. Continues to be impulsive and a safety risk. He still plans to ultimately go home and live with his wife.

References

1. American Physical Therapy Association. *Guide to Physical Therapist Practice*. 2nd ed. Alexandria, VA: APTA; 2003.
2. Agency for Healthcare Research and Quality. Outcomes research (Fact sheet). AHRQ Publication 00-P011. http://www.ahrq.gov/clinic/outfact.htm. Accessed July 8, 2012.
3. Ingersoll GL. Generating evidence through outcomes management. In: Melnyk BM, Fineout-Overholt E, eds. *Evidence-Based Practice in Nursing and Healthcare: A Guide to Best Practice*. Philadelphia, PA: Lippincott Williams & Wilkins; 2005:299-332.
4. Granger CV, Potter PJ, Talavera F, Salcido R, Allen KL, Cailliet R. Quality and outcome measures for rehabilitation programs. http://emedicine.medscape.com/article/317865-overview. Accessed July 8, 2012.
5. Hart DL. What should you expect from the study of clinical outcomes? *J Orthop Sports Phys Ther*. 1998;28:1-2.
6. Jette AM. Outcomes research: shifting the dominant research paradigm in physical therapy. *Phys Ther*. 1995;75:965-970.
7. Finch E, Brooks D, Statford PW, Mayo NE. *Physical Rehabilitation Outcomes Measures*. 2nd ed. Philadelphia, PA: Lippincott Williams & Wilkins; 2002.
8. Resnik L, Liu D, Hart DL, Mor V. Benchmarking physical therapy clinical performance: statistical methods to enhance internal validity when using observational data. *Phys Ther*. 2008;88:1078-1087.
9. Centers for Medicare & Medicaid Services. 2011 Physical Quality Reporting System Measure Specifications Manual for Claims and Registry Reporting of Individual Measures, v5.3. http://www.cms.gov/Medicare/Quality-Initiatives-Patient-Assessment-Instruments/PQRS/downloads/2011_PhysQualRptg_MeasureSpecificationsManual_033111.pdf. Accessed July 15, 2012.
10. Centers for Medicare & Medicaid Services. Physician Quality Reporting System. http://www.cms.gov/Medicare/Quality-Initiatives-Patient-Assessment-Instruments/PQRS/index.html?redirect=/pqrs. Accessed July 15, 2012.
11. Lohr KN. Outcomes measurement: concepts and questions. *Inquiry*. 1988;25:37-50.
12. Wakefield DS. Measuring health care outcomes: more work to do. *J Orthop Sports Phys Ther*. 1998;27:111-113.

Chapter 12

Documentation and Reimbursement

Ralph R. Utzman, PT, MPH, PhD

CHAPTER OUTLINE

CHAPTER OBJECTIVES

Upon completion of this chapter, the reader will be able to:
1. Describe how insurance protects patients from financial risk.
2. List sources of funding for health insurance plans.

Erickson ML, Utzman RR, McKnight R. *Physical Therapy Documentation:*
From Examination to Outcome, Second Edition (pp 125-135).
© 2014 SLACK Incorporated.

3. Outline methods used by insurance companies to control costs.

4. Define prospective payment.

5. Compare different payment models: fee for service, payment per visit or per day, payment per episode, and capitation.

6. List the 4 main "parts" of Medicare and state what types of services are covered by each.

7. Identify the payment methodology used by Medicare in the following settings: outpatient, acute care hospital, inpatient rehabilitation facility, skilled nursing facility, home health.

8. Discuss the importance of gathering registration and insurance information prior to the initiation of care.

9. Name both the current and planned systems for coding patient diagnoses.

10. Name the system used to code for services and procedures.

11. Discuss how coding systems allow for transmission of billing claims from health care providers to insurers.

12. Discuss the importance of documentation for the prevention of claims denials.

13. Describe documentation strategies to prevent claims denials.

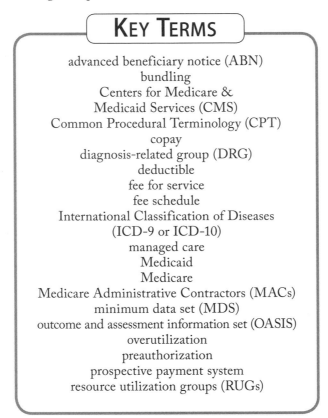

KEY TERMS

advanced beneficiary notice (ABN)
bundling
Centers for Medicare &
Medicaid Services (CMS)
Common Procedural Terminology (CPT)
copay
diagnosis-related group (DRG)
deductible
fee for service
fee schedule
International Classification of Diseases
(ICD-9 or ICD-10)
managed care
Medicaid
Medicare
Medicare Administrative Contractors (MACs)
minimum data set (MDS)
outcome and assessment information set (OASIS)
overutilization
preauthorization
prospective payment system
resource utilization groups (RUGs)

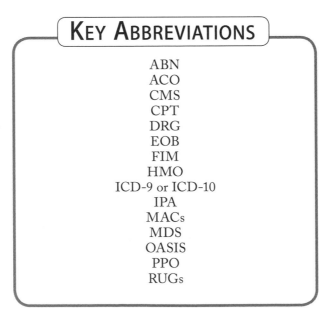

KEY ABBREVIATIONS

ABN
ACO
CMS
CPT
DRG
EOB
FIM
HMO
ICD-9 or ICD-10
IPA
MACs
MDS
OASIS
PPO
RUGs

PT reimbursement is dependent on clear, concise, and accurate documentation. Depending on care setting and payer source, third-party payers consider a combination of factors to determine payment, including patient diagnosis, severity of illness, level of assistance needed, treatment procedures delivered, and outcomes of care. This chapter introduces basic insurance concepts and current and emerging payment models for physical therapy care. Because of Medicare's importance in setting payment policy, this chapter also provides a brief background of Medicare. Finally, this chapter outlines the process for claims submission, including coding systems for diagnoses and procedures.

INSURANCE BASICS

Insurance provides a person with protection from financial risks. Most people do not have enough money in their savings accounts to purchase a new home if their house burns down, or to buy a new car in case of an accident or theft. Homeowner's insurance and auto insurance help cover these costs. Likewise, health insurance protects people from financial catastrophe if they have an illness or an injury.

Insurance provides this financial protection by creating a pool of money that can be used to provide coverage for a large group of people. When a covered event (eg, a fire, a car accident, or an illness) occurs, money from the pool is used to cover the necessary expenses. In the case of home and car insurance, most people pay regular premiums that are added to the pool of money. In the case of health care insurance, most Americans do not pay the premiums that fund their health care insurance. For 45% of the US population, part or all of their premiums are paid by their employers as a benefit of employment.[1] Medicare and Medicaid are public, tax-funded programs that provide insurance coverage for older, retired adults and some younger people who do not have access to employer-sponsored insurance, who make up nearly 30% of the population.[1] About 5% of Americans pay for their own health insurance premiums. The remaining 20% has no health insurance.[1]

Traditionally, insurance plans have paid for health care using an indemnity model similar to car and home insurance. A patient with an indemnity plan would seek care from a health care provider, and then pay for the care delivered. The patient would then seek reimbursement from the insurance company. In more contemporary indemnity plans, the health care provider submits the claim on the patient's behalf and is paid directly by the insurer.

Over the past several decades, the costs of health care in the US have risen dramatically. Although there are many reasons for the rise in costs, insurance insulates patients and providers from the costs of health care. Patients and providers make different choices than they would make if patients paid for health care out of their own pockets, leading to overutilization of services.[2] Managed care is one approach to slowing the rise in costs. In managed care plans, insurance companies have more control over the care delivered to patients. There are many different types of managed care plans, but all use a variety of cost-control mechanisms. These mechanisms are designed to change the behavior of patients and health care providers and facilities.

Managed care plans control individual patient behavior through gatekeeping, cost sharing, or restricting choice. Gatekeeping involves requiring a referral from a primary care physician to see a specialist or to receive certain tests or therapeutic procedures. Cost sharing involves having the patient pay annual deductibles or copays for each visit. With a deductible, the patient is required to pay for a certain amount of care each year (eg, $500) before the health insurance begins to pay. A copay is a fee the patient pays at each visit. For example, a patient may have a $25 copay for each outpatient physical therapy visit. Managed care companies may restrict patient choice by requiring them to seek care from specific doctors, therapists, or hospitals that are part of their network. Other plans may allow patients to seek care from out-of-network providers or facilities if they pay larger copays.

To control the behavior of health care providers, managed care plans develop employment or contractual arrangements with providers. Some health maintenance organizations (HMOs) hire all their health care providers, including physicians, as employees; these are called staff model HMOs. Independent practice associations (IPAs), or preferred provider organizations (PPOs), develop contractual agreements with physicians and other providers who agree to accept negotiated payment rates for delivering care. Managed care plans may also use case management processes to review care and approve payment for services to individual patients. For example, a managed care company may require a physical therapy plan of care to be reviewed for preauthorization before intervention can be provided. Some managed care companies will review documentation periodically during an episode of care to make sure care is being delivered appropriately and efficiently. They may also review payment claims and documentation after an episode of care is complete. If documentation does not demonstrate that appropriate care was provided, the managed care plan will deny reimbursement for part or all of the claim.

Managed care plans influence provider (and patient) behavior, and thus costs of care, by placing limits on the care they will pay for. For example, plans may exclude payment for certain patient diagnoses or treatments. Some plans will limit the number of outpatient therapy visits they will pay for per year. Others may limit the number of therapy procedures they will pay for per visit. Others will place a cap on the dollar amount they will reimburse for therapy per year. Finally, managed care companies can use different payment methodologies to encourage clinicians to limit unnecessary care.

The traditional indemnity model of insurance payment reimburses providers for every single procedure or service they provide. For a patient in the hospital, the insurance company would be billed for every aspirin, wound dressing, and therapy visit the patient receives. In this fee for service model, insurance companies assume the highest financial risk and least control compared with other payment models. Contemporary insurance plans that pay using a fee-for-service model will typically set or negotiate a fee schedule that specifies how much the plan will pay for each individual procedure.

Because the fee for service model is risky for insurers, they have developed various reimbursement models that bundle services together into more affordable packages. Consider the "combo meal" pricing strategy used by many fast-food restaurants. The combo meal prices bundle individual items together at a discounted price. In health care, services can be bundled in several ways. The most common strategies in physical therapy care are bundling by visit, by day, or by episode.

When care is bundled by visits, the insurer pays a set rate for each visit. The provider received the same amount per visit regardless of the number of services or products received during the visit. In inpatient settings, it makes more sense to bundle by day. That is, the insurer will pay a daily fee to the facility regardless of the services the patient receives each day. Payment can also be bundled by an entire episode of care. In this model, the provider receives a lump sum payment for an entire episode of care, such as a hospital stay. Regardless of the length of the episode of care and the intensity of the care provided, the provider or hospital receives the same lump sum payment. These models pose less financial risk for insurance company than fee-for-service payment. Health care providers have more incentive to provide effective and efficient care to keep costs down. Bundled models are often called prospective payment systems because the amount of reimbursement is determined before the episode of care ends.

Another payment model, used primarily by managed care plans, is capitation. In a capitation payment system, the health care provider agrees to provide care for a defined group of people for a set period of time. Capitation payment models pose the least financial risks to insurance companies because care is bundled for an entire group of people over a period of time. The health care provider receives the same amount of money regardless of how many people in the group need care or how the care is provided.

Managed care plans became very popular in the 1990s because of their potential to reduce health care costs and thus reduce insurance premiums paid by individuals, employers, and taxpayers. These various approaches achieved only modest success at slowing the rise in costs. In 2010, President Barack Obama signed the Patient Protection and Affordable Care Act. This law establishes an extensive series of reforms for the US health care system. One section of the PPACA required the CMS to develop a payment model that rewards providers for reducing costs by providing high quality care.[3] As of this writing, the resulting Accountable Care Organization (ACO) model is being tested in several locations around the country.

MORE ABOUT MEDICARE

Medicare is a social insurance program that was established in 1965 to provide health insurance coverage for Americans age 65 years and older, for younger Americans with disabilities and for those with end-stage renal disease.[4]

Congress created the program by enacting Title XVIII of the Social Security Act. At the same time, Congress passed Title XVII, which created Medicaid, to provide insurance coverage for low-income citizens who are younger than 65 years. These laws created a federal agency, now known as CMS, to oversee both programs. To administer the Medicare program, CMS contracts with regional different Medicare administrative contractors (MACs) around the country. The MACs receive, review, and pay Medicare claims for health care services provided in their respective regions.

Medicare has undergone many changes over the years. The original Medicare program was designed to pay for hospital stays and physician visits and operated on an indemnity insurance model. In the early 1970s, outpatient physical therapy was added as a covered benefit. In the 1980s and 1990s, new payment models were established in various care settings. These new payment models have profoundly influenced physical therapy practice, including documentation.

Medicare Part A

Medicare Part A was originally designed to cover inpatient hospital stays. Most patients do not pay a premium to receive Medicare Part A. Over the years, Part A coverage has been expanded to pay for care provided in inpatient rehabilitation hospitals, skilled nursing facilities and subacute care units, and home health agencies. Medicare uses different payment models in each of these care settings.

Acute Care Hospital Reimbursement

Initially, Medicare Part A paid hospitals using a fee for service model of reimbursement. In the 1980s, CMS introduced a prospective payment model in which the hospital receives a lump sum payment based on the patient's diagnosis. Upon discharge, the patient is classified into a diagnosis-related group (DRG) based on his or her diagnosis and severity of illness.[5] The hospital receives a lump sum payment to cover the whole hospital stay (episode) based on the patient's DRG grouping. If the hospital provides efficient care, the hospital keeps the entire lump sum payment, even if the care provided did not cost that much. However, payment will not be increased if the care provided costs more than the lump sum payment. The goal of this payment mechanism is for hospitals to provide care as efficiently as possible and reduce the length of hospital stays. As a result, there has been an increased need for care in postacute care settings.

Inpatient Rehabilitation Facilities

An inpatient rehabilitation facility (IRF) provides comprehensive rehabilitation to patients after serious illness or injury. An IRF can be a freestanding facility or a unit within an acute care hospital. To qualify for IRF admission, a patient must be able to tolerate a minimum of 3 hours of therapy per day.[6] Upon admission to an IRF, a patient is carefully screened and evaluated by a physician.

The patient is then evaluated by an interprofessional team of physical, occupational, and speech therapists; rehabilitation nurses; and orthotist/prosthetists.

Medicare reimburses IRFs using a prospective payment system. The patient's functional status is evaluated by the Functional Independence Measure (FIM) described in Chapter 8. Based on the patient's FIM score, medical diagnosis, comorbidities, and age, the patient is assigned a case mix index.[6] This case mix index determines the payment the IRF will receive for the episode of care. Much like the DRG payment system in acute care hospitals, the episode-based payment provides an incentive for the IRF to provide care in an efficient manner.

Skilled Nursing Facilities and Subacute Care Units

Some hospitalized patients who are not medically stable enough to go home may not need or be able to tolerate the intensity of services offered in an IRF. Skilled nursing facilities (SNFs) can also provide rehabilitation and nursing care to prepare patients to return home. SNFs can be freestanding or they can be units within hospitals or nursing homes. Medicare uses a per-day payment model to reimburse SNF care. Upon admission, each patient is evaluated using a tool called the minimum data set (MDS) and classified into 1 of 66 resource utilization groups (RUGs).[7] The RUG categories are based on the patient's functional status, the services needed (PT, OT, nursing, etc), and a projection of the minutes of therapy the patient will need each week.[7] The patient is reevaluated periodically so that the RUG classification can be adjusted as the patient's status improves. Medicare will typically pay for up to 100 days of SNF care as long as the medical record shows that care is medically necessary, skilled in nature, and results in improved patient function.[7] Medicare pays 100% of the assigned daily reimbursement rate for the first 20 days of an SNF stay. After 20 days in an SNF, the patient pays a copay of 20% of the daily rate.[7]

Home Health Care

After discharge from a hospital, IRF, or SNF, some patients are still in need of skilled therapy or nursing services. Home health agencies send PTs, nurses, and other providers into the patient's home to deliver the necessary care. When a patient receives home health services under Medicare Part A, the patient must be homebound. This means the patient cannot easily leave the home without assistance, although occasional outings (eg, for medical appointments or to attend church) are permitted.[8] The patient is assessed using a comprehensive evaluation tool called the outcome and assessment information set (OASIS).[8] The OASIS tool collects information about the patient's medical condition, functional status, and the amount of care needed by the patient. Based on this information, Medicare pays the home health agency a lump sum payment for the entire home health episode of care.[8]

Medicare Part B

Medicare Part B pays for care provided by physicians and certain outpatient services, including outpatient physical therapy. Unlike Medicare Part A, patients must pay a monthly premium to receive Medicare Part B.[9] The amount of the premium varies based on income and it is adjusted each year.[9] It is possible for a patient to have Medicare Part A, but not Medicare Part B if the patient chooses not to pay the Part B premium.

Medicare Part B pays for physical therapy services using a fee-for-service model. Each procedure (or service) provided by the PT is weighted using a system of relative value units (RVUs). The RVU system takes into account the practice expense, work expense, and malpractice/liability expense of each individual procedure.[10] Each procedure's RVU weight is multiplied by a conversion factor and a geographic adjustment that determines how much the therapist will be paid for the procedure.[10] The RVU payment system is used to develop the Medicare physician fee schedule, which is updated annually.[10]

Because paying by individual procedures can lead to overutilization of services, Medicare has implemented several cost-control mechanisms. First, physical therapy claims are reviewed to make sure the care provided matches the patient's diagnosis and to look for an excessive number of treatment procedures or visits. Second, CMS has instituted a therapy cap, which limits the amount of physical, occupational, and speech therapy a patient can receive each year.[10] This cap is unpopular among patient advocacy groups and rehabilitation professionals because the cap does not take into account the patient's medical condition, functional status, or other individual factors.[11] As a result, various strategies have been used over the past 10 years to allow exceptions to the cap for patients who need additional therapy. CMS is currently evaluating different payment models, such as a per-visit payment system, that may eventually replace the therapy cap and the fee-for-service payment model for outpatient therapy.

Other cost-control mechanisms under Medical Part B include claims reviews and audits. Medicare MACs and auditors may request and review physical therapy documentation to make sure it complies with standards outlined in Chapter 15 of the Medicare Benefit Policy Manual.[12] The manual states that the PT must develop a plan of care for each patient based on the physical therapy examination. The examination must include standard functional measures such as those described in Chapter 8.[12] The initial plan of care must then be reviewed and certified (signed) by a physician.[12] The plan of care must be recertified by a physician at least once every 90 days, or sooner if indicated in the original plan of care.[12] The manuals also require that the PT reassess the patient at least once over 10 visits and report on the patient's progress related to the initial plan of care.[12] If a PTA is involved in the patient's care, the PTA may document interim treatment notes, but the supervising therapist is responsible for documenting the initial examination and plan of care, subsequent progress reports, and a discharge summary.[12]

Medicare Part C

The Balanced Budget Act of 1997 created the option for Medicare recipients to enroll in managed care plans in place of traditional Medicare Parts A and B. Originally called "Medicare+Choice" plans, these managed-care products are delivered by privately managed-care organizations. Now known as "Medicare Advantage," these plans became popular with many seniors because they may provide coverage for services not covered under traditional Medicare, such as expanded prescription drug coverage, dental and vision benefits, and health club memberships. Medicare pays the managed care plan a monthly fee and many Medicare Advantage enrollees also pay a monthly premium.[13] The Medicare Advantage plans operate just like other managed-care plans described earlier in the chapter.

Medicare Part D

Part D was added to Medicare in 2006 to provide coverage for prescription drugs. Part D allows Medicare recipients to enroll in private prescription insurance plans or a Medicare Part C plan that offers coverage for prescription drugs.

PROCESSES FOR MANAGING REIMBURSEMENT CLAIMS

As noted earlier in the chapter, Medicare is one of many third-party payers of health care in the United States. However, Medicare often serves as a useful model for learning about reimbursement. Many other insurance companies and plans model their reimbursement policies after Medicare. In some settings, such as skilled nursing and home health, Medicare is the most common payer source.

Regardless of whether the patient has social insurance like Medicare, employer-sponsored insurance, or privately purchased insurance, the process for submitting claims for reimbursement is very similar. The process begins before care is delivered to verify the patient's insurance benefits. After care is provided and documented, information about the encounter is converted into codes that are entered onto a paper billing form or transmitted to an electronic billing system. The bill is then mailed or transmitted to the insurance plan for payment. This process is described in more detail in the remainder of the chapter.

Before Care Is Delivered

When a patient is referred to outpatient physical therapy, or admitted to an inpatient facility, the patient is registered. Registration involves collecting demographic, contact, and insurance information about the patient. If a patient has previously received care at the same facility, the registration process may simply involve updating information currently on file. When registering a patient, you should make a photocopy of the patient's insurance card. The back of the card may include important information, so you should copy both sides. Any documents that accompany the patient, such as written referrals or copies of relevant medical records from other providers, should be collected and placed in the patient's chart. If a patient is covered by more than one insurance plan, you should get information for all the plans.

Next, the patient's insurance benefits should be verified. If your clinic or practice has a contractual agreement with the patient's insurance company, your billing office should have information for completing this step. If not, use the information from the patient's insurance card to contact the insurance plan for more information. It is important to verify insurance companies in case the patient's coverage has been cancelled or expired. Also, if the patient is covered by more than one insurance plan, you will need to determine which one will be the primary payer.

Besides verifying that the patient has insurance coverage, you also need to find out what information is required for coverage of the services you plan to provide and if there are any services that the insurance company excludes. In many settings, insurance plans will require the provider to submit referrals, examination results, or other documentation in order to preauthorize payment before care is provided.

Following Initiation of Care

After care is initiated, information about the patient and the care provided needs to be converted to a format that can be transmitted to the insurance company. This process is called coding. Both the patient's diagnosis and the treatment provided are typically converted into codes.

Diagnosis Coding

The World Health Organization (WHO; developed the ICF model discussed in earlier chapters) also publishes a coding system for diseases, injuries, and other health conditions. This coding system is known as the International Classification of Diseases (ICD). In the United States, health care providers have used the 9th edition of this coding system, ICD-9, for 30 years. In ICD-9, diseases and injuries are represented by a series of numeric codes. An ICD-9 code includes a minimum of 3 and a maximum of 5 digits. The first 3 digits represent the health condition itself and are followed by a decimal. Two more digits can be added after the digit to provide clarification, such as describing which part of the body is involved.

For example, ICD-9 code 715 represents the health condition osteoarthritis. This diagnosis is very broad because osteoarthritis can involve one or more joints.[14] According to the ICD-9 code set, 2 more digits can be added to specify which joint is being treated and whether that joint is the primary site of joint involvement. Therefore, the 5-digit code 715.15 indicates that the patient has osteoarthritis (the first 3 digits), that the joint being treated is the primary site of involvement (the 4th digit), and that the joint being treated is the patient's knee.[14]

Therapists can find ICD-9 codes in a number of places. A CD-ROM of the entire ICD-9 code set can be purchased from the US government's printing office for a nominal fee. The Internet address for ordering is http://bookstore.gpo.gov/actions/GetPublication.do?stock number=017-022-01616-8. The *Guide for Physical Therapist Practice* provides partial lists of ICD-9 codes organized by practice pattern. The list provided in the *Guide* is not a complete listing; the *Guide* may not provide the necessary 4th and 5th digits. Therefore, you should use a more complete list of ICD-9 codes for looking up codes for billing. The APTA also publishes coding manuals designed for PTs that include diagnosis and procedure codes.

On October 1, 2014, all health care providers in the United States will be required to use the newer ICD-10 code set.[15] This coding system uses numbers and letters in codes that include 3 to 7 characters. The ICD-10 code set has been used in some other countries since the 1990s. The ICD-10 codes allow more specific coding than ICD-9 and uses more contemporary terminology.[16] It is expected that ICD-10 will allow improved accuracy of coding and tracking of submitted insurance claims.[16] Information on ordering manuals of the US version of ICD-10, as well as details on the transition to ICD-10, are available on the US Centers for Disease Control and Prevention Web site at http://www.cdc.gov/nchs/icd/icd10.htm.

Coding for Procedures

In many settings, the Common Procedural Terminology (CPT) coding system is used to describe treatments provided to patients. The American Medical Association (AMA) publishes and copyrights the CPT code set. Coding manuals can be purchased directly from the AMA or from book retailers. Other publishers offer coding manuals tailored to specific professions or care settings.

CPT codes consist of 7 numeric digits. For example, CPT code 97001 is used to indicate that a physical therapy evaluation was performed.[17] Table 12-1 lists many of the codes PTs use frequently. Many of the codes stipulate that the provider must provide direct one-on-one contact with the patient throughout the treatment period. Many codes are "timed" codes that specify treatment should be provided in 15-minute increments. According to the CPT coding manual, a 15-minute "unit" can be billed when at least half of the 15-minute time frame has elapsed.[17] If the treatment lasts more than 15 minutes, additional units can be billed once the halfway point of the next unit has been passed.[17] For example:

> 1 unit = at least 8 minutes of treatment provided
> 2 units = at least 23 minutes of treatment provided
> 3 units = at least 38 minutes of treatment provided
> 4 units = at least 53 minutes of treatment provided

Sometimes, a CPT code alone does not adequately describe the services provided to this patient. In these cases, modifiers can be added. Modifiers are 2-character codes that can include both numbers and letters. For example, the modifier -GP added to the CPT code 97001 indicates that the physical therapy examination was performed by a PT. Another common example is modifier -59.[14] There are therapeutic procedures that are similar and may overlap with each other. Aquatic therapy involves exercise in the water. If a PT performed aquatic exercises with a patient, it would be inappropriate to bill both CPT codes 97110 (therapeutic exercise)[17] and 97113 (aquatic therapy)[17] for that treatment. However, if a therapist instructs a patient in land-based exercises for 15 minutes, then spends another 15 minutes on aquatic exercise, it would be appropriate to code and bill for both of these procedures. The therapist would add the -59 modifier to indicate that the 2 procedures were provided to the patient at distinctly different times.

As you document patient care, keep in mind that the medical record will often be compared with the codes (both diagnostic and procedure codes) listed on the insurance claim form. Your documentation must support the ICD and CPT codes listed on the claim.

Other Coding Systems

Besides ICD and CPT coding systems, other systems have emerged to describe patients and the care provided to them. In the SNF setting described earlier, the data collected on the MDS assessment tool are converted to codes that are transmitted to the MAC that handles the claim. Similarly, data collected on the OASIS tool in home health are converted to codes for billing and review purposes.

Billing

Once data regarding the patient and the care provided to the patient are translated into codes, these codes are recorded on a claim form or entered into an electronic billing system. Most use standard formats for submission of billing claims. The CMS-1500 form was developed by CMS and is now widely used by most insurers to pay for outpatient services provided in private offices.[18] Outpatient services offered by hospitals and other institution-based clinics typically use a UB-04 form.[19] Both of these forms collect information gathered during the patient registration process as well as diagnosis and treatment information in the form of ICD and CPT codes. These forms are then submitted, either by mail or electronically, to the insurance company (or regional MAC in the case of Medicare) for reimbursement.

Claims Denials and Appeals

After you submit a health insurance claim, the insurer reviews and processes the claim. If there are problems with the claim, the insurer may deny payment. The insurer typically sends a notice of the denial, called an Explanation of Benefits (EOB), to the patient and the provider. If the claim was denied for technical errors (eg, missing information on the claim form, minor coding problems), the provider can fix the problems and resubmit. If the claim was denied for a

Table 12-1
Common Procedural Terminology Codes
Commonly Used by Physical Therapists*

Author's Note: This brief list is a sample of CPT codes that may be used by physical therapists. For a more comprehensive listing, please consult a CPT coding manual available from the American Medical Association. Individual payers may reimburse some codes but not others. You should check with the payer to determine coverage.

Code	Description	Timed Code?
Evaluation Procedures *Author's note: These codes may not be billed by a PTA. Code 97001 is typically used at the first PT visit. Code 97002 should be used when the therapist re-evaluates the patient and revises the plan of care because of a significant change in the patient's status. 97002 is typically not used for ongoing reassessment of the patient that occurs as part of a routine visit.*		
97001	Physical Therapy Evaluation	No
97002	Physical Therapy Reevaluation	No
Unattended Therapeutic Modalities *Author's note: For those modalities, the PT (or PTA under PT supervision) sets up the modality, provides patient instruction, and provides ongoing supervision during the treatment.*		
97010	Hot packs/cold packs	No
97012	Mechanical traction	No
97014	Electrical stimulation	No
97016	Vasopneumatic devices	No
97018	Paraffin bath	No
97022	Whirlpool	No
97024	Diathermy	No
Constant Attendance Therapeutic Modalities *Author's note: For these modalities, the PT (or PTA under PT supervision) sets up the modality and provides patient instruction. The PT (or PTA) must provide direct, one-on-one patient contact throughout the procedure. These codes are timed in 15-minute increments.*		
97032	Electrical stimulation	Yes
97033	Iontophoresis	Yes
97034	Contrast baths	Yes
97035	Ultrasound	Yes
97036	Hubbard tank	Yes
Therapeutic Procedures *Author's note: For all except 97150, the PT (or PTA) must provide direct, one-on-one patient contact throughout the procedure; codes are timed in 15-minute increments. Code 97150 is untimed, and can be billed only once per visit.*		
97110	Therapeutic exercise (strength, endurance, flexibility)	Yes
97112	Neuromuscular reeducation (movement, balance, coordination, proprioception)	Yes
97113	Aquatic therapy	Yes
97116	Gait training	Yes
97124	Massage	Yes
97140	Manual therapy techniques	Yes
97150	Group, 2 or more individuals	No
97530	Therapeutic activities	Yes
97533	Sensory integration	Yes
97535	Self-care/home management	Yes

*CPT copyright 2012 American Medical Association. All rights reserved.

coverage issue (eg, the documentation does not demonstrate medical necessity or provision of skilled service; the treatment provided or health condition is excluded by the insurance plan), the payer and/or patient may file an appeal.

You should appeal a claim denial if you believe the care you provided met the coverage requirements of the insurance plan and that the documentation proves you provided reasonable, necessary skilled care. Medicare's appeal process is outlined on the CMS Web site (http://www.cms.gov/Outreach-and-Education/Medicare-Learning-Network-MLN/MLNProducts/downloads/medicareappealsprocess.pdf). Managed care, employer-based, and private health plans should also have appeals processes. You can often find these on the insurance companies' Web sites, in the provider contract agreement, or by contacting the insurer directly.

Appealing a claim denial takes time, meaning you may not get paid for services provided for several months. Appeals also require time and attention from the clinician and billing staff. Therefore, it is always better to prevent a denial than to file an appeal. Some strategies for preventing denials:

- **Make sure your documentation and billing are accurate and consistent.** It is not uncommon for payers to request copies of your documentation for review. Your documentation must be complete and support the treatment provided. Never change your documentation after it is complete. Although it may

be tempting to go back and add details later, if you change a note after copies are already shared with insurers, it could be perceived as fraud.

- **Carefully read and understand the CPT code descriptions.** CPT coding manuals provide descriptors to help determine which code is the best to use for a specific procedure or service. For example, CPT codes 97110 and 97112 are both listed as "therapeutic procedures."[17] The description for code 97110 clarifies that this code should be used for therapeutic exercises to improve strength, endurance, range of motion, or flexibility.[17] The description for code 97112 states this code should be used for exercises related to balance, coordination, and proprioception.[17] Also, when using timed CPT codes, make sure the treatment times listed for each procedure and the total treatment time are accurate (see Chapter 8).

- **Be aware of insurance exclusions and limitations.** If you provide treatment to a patient that you feel the insurer will not cover, you should discuss this with your patient before providing the service. In some cases, if the patient chooses to receive the treatment after being notified that insurance will not pay for it, the patient may be billed directly for the service. See Example 12-1.[20]

Example 12-1. Services That Are Excluded or Limited by an Insurance Plan

Insurance plans exclude or limit services to make sure that they pay only for services that are effective, reasonable, and necessary for the patient's condition. Sometimes, patients will choose to receive excluded or limited services anyway. Patients must be fully informed of their financial obligations if they choose services that are not expected to be covered by their insurance.

In some instances, if a patient chooses to receive an excluded procedure, you may be able to bill the patient for the services directly if the patient is notified in writing in advance. Medicare requires use of a standard informed consent form, known as an advanced beneficiary notice (ABN) form, when you expect a reimbursement claim to be denied. CMS has posted the ABN form for download at http://www.cms.gov/Medicare/Medicare-General-Information/BNI/downloads/cmsr131g.pdf.

One use of the ABN occurs when you provide a service that is typically covered by Medicare, but you believe it will be denied because it's not reasonable or necessary for a particular patient.

Example: Patient A has been receiving therapy 3 times per week for a period of 6 weeks. She has improved and is independent with her home exercise program. The therapist determines that reducing visit frequency to once per

week for monitoring and progressing the home program is appropriate. The patient disagrees and would like to continue attending 3 visits per week.

Having the patient sign an ABN is required in this case because the PT feels that 3 visits per week are not reasonable or necessary and expects Medicare to deny payment for this visit frequency.

If the patient chooses to continue therapy 3 times per week, the patient checks the appropriate box on the form and signs it. The therapist then delivers the care and submits the claim to Medicare. If Medicare does indeed deny to pay the claim because the frequency of visits is deemed excessive, the therapist may then bill the patient directly for the denied visits.

The ABN form is specific to Medicare Parts A and B. When working with patients who have other forms of insurance (private, employer based, or Medicare Advantage), you should contact the insurer directly and inquire about their policies.

Reference: Centers for Medicare & Medicaid Services. Advanced Beneficiary Notice of Noncoverage (ABN), Form CMS-R-131 Updated Manual Instructions. CMS Transmittal 2480. http://www.cms.gov/Regulations-and-Guidance/Guidance/Transmittals/Downloads/R2480CP.pdf. Accessed November 2, 2012.

- **Make documentation understandable for professionals as well as the lay public.** To be understandable, documentation must be legible. If you write notes by hand, your penmanship must be easy to read. Illegible notes frustrate readers who may not be able to decipher important information that supports the insurance claim. Illegible notes can also lead to medical errors and jeopardize patient safety.

  Another important way to make documentation understandable is to limit abbreviations and avoid jargon. Even if a fellow therapist can read and understand your notes, other readers who do not have the same professional training may not be familiar with the terminology and abbreviations we use every day. This makes it hard for readers to follow your decision-making process and to determine whether the patient received necessary skilled care. Use only standard abbreviations and write your documentation with the lay person in mind.

- **Show skill and integrate CPT code terminology when describing interventions in the Objective section and plan of care.** General descriptions of interventions that do not include the parameters of treatment do not demonstrate skilled care. Remember to describe how your involvement was necessary (see Chapter 8 for an example). Also, consider using CPT code language in our descriptions. For example, use the words "gait training" instead of "ambulation."

- **Cultivate good documentation habits.** The life of a PT is hectic and creating quality documentation can be time consuming. Unfortunately, some clinicians take "shortcuts" when documenting that may seem efficient at the time but can lead to claims denials later on. Taking shortcuts can lead to inaccurate documents or documents that fail to demonstrate the need for services, provision of skilled care, or patient progress.

Documentation is most accurate when it is completed during or immediately following care delivery. You may forget important details if hours (or days) pass between care delivery and documentation. Although not every note can be completed during the treatment session, you should always complete documentation the same day care was delivered. Besides inviting claims denials, incomplete and inaccurate notes can present patient safety and legal liability risks (see Chapter 3).

Be careful to avoid using phrases that tell the reader nothing. For example, writing "Tolerated treatment well" in the Assessment section does not provide any information about how the patient actually tolerated treatment. Did the patient report less pain or fatigue? Was the patient able to tolerate more exercises or activity? Did the patient ask questions, and how did you answer these questions? Paint a picture for the reader to illustrate the patient's response to treatment and any progress made so your decision-making process is clear.

Similarly, avoid writing phrases such as "Continue as above" or "Follow" in the Plan section of the note. Readers will look to the plan of care to find out how you are moving the patient's treatment along over time. Use of these phrases does not show progress.

Review Questions

1. How does insurance protect patients from financial risk? How might this protection impact patients' choices regarding their health care? How might this protection impact the behavior of health care providers?

2. What is the difference between a premium and a copayment? How might these mechanisms impact patient behavior with respect to seeking health care?

3. What is meant by the term managed care?

4. How does Medicare pay for care delivered in acute care hospitals? Inpatient rehab facilities? Skilled nursing facilities? Home health agencies? Outpatient physical therapy clinics?

5. What is the difference between ICD codes and CPT codes?

6. What steps can you take to reduce the risk that insurance claims will be denied?

Instead, clearly document the interventions provided in the Objective section (see Chapter 8) and, in the Plan section, tell the reader what you will be doing with the patient at the next visit.

APPLICATION EXERCISES

1. Review an interim/daily note for an outpatient (it could be a patient either you or a colleague treated). From the description of the interventions provided, determine which CPT codes should be used on the reimbursement claim form.

2. Review an initial examination note written by a classmate, clinical instructor, or colleague. Critique the note from an insurance company's perspective. Share your feedback with the author of the note.

3. In the clinic, choose a patient whose care you documented. Working with the clinic staff, follow the reimbursement claim from filing to final payment. During the process, take note of how many people had access to the medical record. Was payment obtained on the first attempt? How could documentation be improved?

REFERENCES

1. Kaiser Family Foundation. Health coverage & uninsured—facts at a glance. http://www.statehealthfacts.org/comparecat.jsp?cat=3&rgn=6&rgn=1. Accessed November 2, 2012.

2. Rasmussen B. Principles of insurance. In: *Reimbursement and Fiscal Management in Rehabilitation*. Alexandria, VA: American Physical Therapy Association; 1995:48-62.

3. US Department of Health and Human Services. Affordable care act to improve quality of care for people with Medicare. http://www.hhs.gov/news/press/2011pres/03/20110331a.html. Accessed November 2, 2012.

4. Centers for Medicare & Medicaid Services. What is Medicare? http://www.medicare.gov/sign-up-change-plans/decide-how-to-get-medicare/whats-medicare/what-is-medicare.html. Accessed November 2, 2012.

5. Medicare Payment Advisory Committee. Hospital acute inpatient services payment system. http://www.medpac.gov/documents/MedPAC_Payment_Basics_12_hospital.pdf. Accessed November 2, 2012.

6. Medicare Payment Advisory Committee. Inpatient rehabilitation facilities payment system. http://www.medpac.gov/documents/MedPAC_Payment_Basics_12_IRF.pdf. Accessed November 2, 2012.

7. Medicare Payment Advisory Committee. Skilled nursing facility services payment system. http://www.medpac.gov/documents/MedPAC_Payment_Basics_12_SNF.pdf. Accessed November 2, 2012.

8. Medicare Payment Advisory Committee. Home health care services payment system. http://www.medpac.gov/documents/MedPAC_Payment_Basics_12_HHA.pdf. Accessed November 2, 2012.

9. Centers for Medicare & Medicaid Services. Part B costs. http://medicare.gov/your-medicare-costs/part-b-costs/part-b-costs.html. Accessed November 2, 2012.

10. Medicare Payment Advisory Committee. Outpatient therapy services payment system. http://www.medpac.gov/documents/MedPAC_Payment_Basics_12_OPT.pdf. Accessed November 2, 2012.

11. Navaro C. Be my Valentine? Coalition to Congress: Show your love for seniors by protecting therapy services. http://www.apta.org/uploadedFiles/APTAorg/Advocacy/Federal/Legislative_Issues/Therapy_Cap/TherapyCapCoaltionUrgesCongresstoProtectServices.pdf. Accessed November 2, 2012.

12. Centers for Medicare & Medicaid Services. Covered medical and other health services. *Medicare Benefit Policy Manual*. Publication 100-02. http://www.cms.gov/Regulations-and-Guidance/Guidance/Manuals/downloads/bp102c15.pdf. Accessed November 2, 2012.

13. Medicare Payment Advisory Committee. Medicare advantage program payment system. http://www.medpac.gov/documents/MedPAC_Payment_Basics_12_MA.pdf. Accessed November 2, 2012.

14. American Physical Therapy Association. *Coding and Payment Guide for the Physical Therapist*. St. Louis, MO: Ingenix; 2009.

15. Centers for Medicare & Medicaid Services. ICD-10. http://www.cms.gov/Medicare/Coding/ICD10/index.html. Accessed November 1, 2012.

16. Centers for Medicare & Medicaid Services. ICD-10-CM/PCS: An introduction. http://www.cms.gov/Medicare/Coding/ICD10/downloads/ICD-10Overview.pdf. Accessed November 2, 2012.

17. American Medical Association. *CPT 2011: Standard Edition*. Chicago, IL: American Medical Association; 2011.

18. Centers for Medicare & Medicaid Services. Form CMS-1500 at a glance. http://www.cms.gov/Outreach-and-Education/Medicare-Learning-Network-MLN/MLNProducts/downloads/form_cms-1500_fact_sheet.pdf. Accessed November 2, 2012.

19. Centers for Medicare & Medicaid Services. UB-04 overview. http://www.cms.gov/Outreach-and-Education/Medicare-Learning-Network-MLN/MLNProducts/downloads/ub04_fact_sheet.pdf. Accessed November 2, 2012.

20. Centers for Medicare & Medicaid Services. Advanced beneficiary notice of noncoverage (ABN), form CMS-R-131 updated manual instructions. http://www.cms.gov/Regulations-and-Guidance/Guidance/Transmittals/Downloads/R2480CP.pdf. Accessed November 2, 2012.

Guidelines: Physical Therapy Documentation of Patient/Client Management

Bod G03-05-16-41 [Amended BOD 02-02-16-20; BOD 11-01-06-10; BOD 03-01-16-51; BOD 03-00-22-54; BOD 03-99-14-41; BOD 11-98-19-69; BOD 03-97-27-69; BOD 03-95-23-61; BOD 11-94-33-107; BOD 06-93-09-13; Initial BOD 03-93-21-55] [Guideline]

PREAMBLE

The American Physical Therapy Association (APTA) is committed to meeting the physical therapy needs of society, to meeting the needs and interests of its members, and to developing and improving the art and science of physical therapy, including practice, education and research. To help meet these responsibilities, APTA's Board of Directors has approved the following guidelines for physical therapy documentation. It is recognized that these guidelines do not reflect all of the unique documentation requirements associated with the many specialty areas within the physical therapy profession. Applicable for both hand-written and electronic documentation systems, these guidelines are intended to be used as a foundation for the development of more specific documentation guidelines in clinical areas, while at the same time providing guidance for the physical therapy profession across all practice settings. Documentation may also need to address additional regulatory or payer requirements.

Finally, be aware that these guidelines are intended to address documentation of patient/client management, not to describe the provision of physical therapy services. Other APTA documents, including APTA Standards of Practice for Physical Therapy, Code of Ethics and Guide for Professional Conduct, and the *Guide to Physical Therapist Practice*, address provision of physical therapy services and patient/client management.

APTA POSITION ON DOCUMENTATION

Documentation Authority for Physical Therapy Services

Physical therapy examination, evaluation, diagnosis, prognosis, and plan of care (including interventions) shall be documented, dated, and authenticated by the physical therapist who performs the service. Interventions provided by the physical therapist or selected interventions provided by the physical therapist assistant under the direction and supervision of the physical therapist are documented, dated, and authenticated by the physical therapist or, when permissible by law, the physical therapist assistant.

Erickson ML, Utzman RR, McKnight R. *Physical Therapy Documentation: From Examination to Outcome, Second Edition* (pp 137-145).
© 2014 SLACK Incorporated.

Other notations or flow charts are considered a component of the documented record but do not meet the requirements of documentation in or of themselves.

Students in physical therapist or physical therapist assistant programs may document when the record is additionally authenticated by the physical therapist or, when permissible by law, documentation by physical therapist assistant students may be authenticated by a physical therapist assistant.

OPERATIONAL DEFINITIONS

Guidelines

APTA defines a "guideline" as a statement of advice.

Authentication

The process used to verify that an entry is complete, accurate, and final. Indications of authentication can include original written signatures and computer "signatures" on secured electronic record systems only.

The following describes the main documentation elements of patient/client management: 1) initial examination/evaluation, 2) visit/encounter, 3) reexamination, and 4) discharge or discontinuation summary.

Initial Examination/Evaluation

Documentation of the initial encounter is typically called the "initial examination," "initial evaluation," or "initial examination/evaluation." Completion of the initial examination/evaluation is typically completed in one visit, but may occur over more than one visit.

Documentation elements for the initial examination/evaluation include the following:

Examination: Includes data obtained from the history, systems review, and tests and measures.

Evaluation: Evaluation is a thought process that may not include formal documentation. It may include documentation of the assessment of the data collected in the examination and identification of problems pertinent to patient/client management.

Diagnosis: Indicates level of impairment, activity limitation, and participation restriction determined by the physical therapist. May be indicated by selecting one or more preferred practice patterns from the *Guide to Physical Therapist Practice*.

Prognosis: Provides documentation of the predicted level of improvement that might be attained through intervention and the amount of time required to reach that level. Prognosis is typically not a separate documentation element, but the components are included as part of the plan of care.

Plan of care: Typically stated in general terms, includes goals, interventions planned, proposed frequency and duration, and discharge plans.

Visit/Encounter

Documentation of a visit or encounter, often called a progress note or daily note, documents sequential implementation of the plan of care established by the physical therapist, including changes in patient/client status and variations and progressions of specific interventions used. Also may include specific plans for the next visit or visits.

Reexamination

Documentation of reexamination includes data from repeated or new examination elements and is provided to evaluate progress and to modify or redirect intervention.

Discharge or Discontinuation Summary

Documentation is required following conclusion of the current episode in the physical therapy intervention sequence, to summarize progression toward goals and discharge plans.

GENERAL GUIDELINES

Documentation is required for every visit/encounter.

- All documentation must comply with the applicable jurisdictional/regulatory requirements.

- All handwritten entries shall be made in ink and will include original signatures. Electronic entries are made with appropriate security and confidentiality provisions.

- Charting errors should be corrected by drawing a single line through the error and initialing and dating the chart or through the appropriate mechanism for electronic documentation that clearly indicates that a change was made without deletion of the original record.

- All documentation must include adequate identification of the patient/client and the physical therapist or physical therapist assistant:

  - The patient's/client's full name and identification number, if applicable, must be included on all official documents.

  - All entries must be dated and authenticated with the provider's full name and appropriate designation:

    - Documentation of examination, evaluation, diagnosis, prognosis, plan of care, and discharge summary must be authenticated by the physical therapist who provided the service.

    - Documentation of intervention in visit/encounter notes must be authenticated by the physical therapist or physical therapist assistant who provided the service.

    - Documentation by physical therapist or physical therapist assistant graduates or other physical therapists and physical therapist assistants pending receipt of an unrestricted license shall be authenticated by a licensed physical therapist, or, when permissible by law, documentation by physical therapist assistant graduates may be authenticated by a physical therapist assistant.

    - Documentation by students (SPT/SPTA) in physical therapist or physical therapist assistant programs must be additionally authenticated by the physical therapist or, when permissible by law, documentation by physical therapist assistant students may be authenticated by a physical therapist assistant.

- Documentation should include the referral mechanism by which physical therapy services are initiated. Examples include:

  - Self-referral/direct access

  - Request for consultation from another practitioner

- Documentation should include indication of no shows and cancellations.

INITIAL EXAMINATION/EVALUATION

Examination (History, Systems Review, and Tests and Measures)

History:

   Documentation of history may include the following:

- General demographics

- Social history

- Employment/work (Job/School/Play)

- Growth and development

- Living environment

- General health status (self-report, family report, caregiver report)

- Social/health habits (past and current)

- Family history

- Medical/surgical history

- Current condition(s)/Chief complaint(s)

- Functional status and activity level

- Medications

- Other clinical tests

Systems Review:
  Documentation of systems review may include gathering data for the following systems:
  - Cardiovascular/pulmonary
    - Blood Pressure
    - Edema
    - Heart Rate
    - Respiratory Rate
  - Integumentary
    - Pliability (texture)
    - Presence of scar formation
    - Skin color
    - Skin integrity
  - Musculoskeletal
    - Gross range of motion
    - Gross strength
    - Gross symmetry
    - Height
    - Weight
  - Neuromuscular
    - Gross coordinated movement (eg, balance, locomotion, transfers, and transitions)
    - Motor function (motor control, motor learning)
  Documentation of systems review may also address communication ability, affect, cognition, language, and learning style:
  - Ability to make needs known
  - Consciousness
  - Expected emotional/behavioral responses
  - Learning preferences (eg, education needs, learning barriers)
  - Orientation (person, place, time)

Tests and Measures:
  Documentation of tests and measures may include findings for the following categories:
  - Aerobic Capacity/Endurance
    Examples of examination findings include:
    - Aerobic capacity during functional activities
    - Aerobic capacity during standardized exercise test protocols
    - Cardiovascular signs and symptoms in response to increased oxygen demand with exercise or activity
    - Pulmonary signs and symptoms in response to increased oxygen demand with exercise or activity
  - Anthropometric Characteristics
    Examples of examination findings include:
    - Body composition
    - Body dimensions
    - Edema
  - Arousal, attention, and cognition
    Examples of examination findings include:
    - Arousal and attention
    - Cognition
    - Communication
    - Consciousness
    - Motivation
    - Orientation to time, person, place, and situation
    - Recall

- Assistive and adaptive devices

  Examples of examination findings include:
  - Assistive or adaptive devices and equipment use during functional activities
  - Components, alignment, fit, and ability to care for the assistive or adaptive devices and equipment
  - Remediation of impairments, activity limitations and participation restrictions with use of assistive or adaptive devices and equipment
  - Safety during use of assistive or adaptive devices and equipment

- Circulation (Arterial, Venous, Lymphatic)

  Examples of examination findings include:
  - Cardiovascular signs
  - Cardiovascular symptoms
  - Physiological responses to position change

- Cranial and Peripheral Nerve Integrity

  Examples of examination findings include:
  - Electrophysiological integrity
  - Motor distribution of the cranial nerves
  - Motor distribution of the peripheral nerves
  - Response to neural provocation
  - Response to stimuli, including auditory, gustatory, olfactory, pharyngeal, vestibular, and visual
  - Sensory distribution of the cranial nerves
  - Sensory distribution of the peripheral nerves

- Environmental, Home, and Work (Job/School/Play) Barriers

  Examples of examination findings include:
  - Current and potential barriers
  - Physical space and environment

- Ergonomics and Body mechanics

  Examples of examination findings for ergonomics include:
  - Dexterity and coordination during work
  - Functional capacity and performance during work actions, tasks, or activities
  - Safety in work environments
  - Specific work conditions or activities
  - Tools, devices, equipment, and work-stations related to work actions, tasks, or activities

  Examples of examination findings for body mechanics include:
  - Body mechanics during self-care, home management, work, community, or leisure actions, tasks, or activities

- Gait, locomotion, and balance

  Examples of examination findings include:
  - Balance during functional activities with or without the use of assistive, adaptive, orthotic, protection, supportive, or prosthetic devices or equipment
  - Balance (dynamic and static) with or without the use of assistive, adaptive, orthotic, protective, supportive, or prosthetic devices or equipment
  - Gait and locomotion during functional activities with or without the use of assistive, adaptive, orthotic, protective, supportive, or prosthetic devices or equipment
  - Gait and locomotion with or without the use of assistive, adaptive, orthotic, protective, supportive, or prosthetic devices or equipment
  - Safety during gait, locomotion, and balance

- Integumentary Integrity

  Examples of examination findings include:
  Associated skin:
  - Activities, positioning, and postures that produce or relieve trauma to the skin
  - Assistive, adaptive, orthotic, protective, supportive, or prosthetic devices and equipment that may produce or relieve trauma to the skin
  - Skin characteristics

- Wound
  - Activities, positioning, and postures that aggravate the wound or scar or that produce or relieve trauma
  - Burn
  - Signs of infection
  - Wound characteristics
  - Wound scar tissue characteristics
- Joint Integrity and Mobility

  Examples of examination findings include:
  - Joint integrity and mobility
  - Joint play movements
  - Specific body parts
- Motor Function

  Examples of examination findings include:
  - Dexterity, coordination, and agility
  - Electrophysiological integrity
  - Hand function
  - Initiation, modification, and control of movement patterns and voluntary postures
- Muscle Performance

  Examples of examination findings include:
  - Electrophysiological integrity
  - Muscle strength, power, and endurance
  - Muscle strength, power, and endurance during functional activities
  - Muscle tension
- Neuromotor development and sensory integration

  Examples of examination findings include:
  - Acquisition and evolution of motor skills
  - Oral motor function, phonation, and speech production
  - Sensorimotor integration
- Orthotic, protective, and supportive devices

  Examples of examination findings include:
  - Components, alignment, fit, and ability to care for the orthotic, protective, and supportive devices and equipment
  - Orthotic, protective, and supportive devices and equipment use during functional activities
  - Remediation of impairments, activity limitations, and participation restrictions with use of orthotic, protective, and supportive devices and equipment
  - Safety during use of orthotic, protective, and supportive devices and equipment
- Pain

  Examples of examination findings include:
  - Pain, soreness, and nocioception
  - Pain in specific body parts
- Posture

Examples of examination findings include:
  - Postural alignment and position (dynamic)
  - Postural alignment and position (static)
  - Specific body parts
- Prosthetic requirements

  Examples of examination findings include:
  - Components, alignment, fit, and ability to care for prosthetic device
  - Prosthetic device use during functional activities
  - Remediation of impairments, activity limitations, and participation restrictions with use of the prosthetic device
  - Residual limb or adjacent segment
  - Safety during use of the prosthetic device

- Range of motion (including muscle length)

  Examples of examination findings include:
  - Functional ROM
  - Joint active and passive movement
  - Muscle length, soft tissue extensibility, and flexibility

- Reflex integrity

  Examples of examination findings include:
  - Deep reflexes
  - Electrophysiological integrity
  - Postural reflexes and reactions, including righting, equilibrium, and protective reactions
  - Primitive reflexes and reactions
  - Resistance to passive stretch
  - Superficial reflexes and reactions

- Self-care and home management (including activities of daily living and instrumental activities of daily living)

  Examples of examination findings include:
  - Ability to gain access to home environments
  - Ability to perform self-care and home management activities with or without assistive, adaptive, orthotic, protective, supportive, or prosthetic devices and equipment
  - Safety in self-care and home management activities and environments

- Sensory integrity

  Examples of examination findings include:
  - Combined/cortical sensations
  - Deep sensations
  - Electrophysiological integrity

- Ventilation and respiration

  Examples of examination findings include:
  - Pulmonary signs of respiration/gas exchange
  - Pulmonary signs of ventilatory function
  - Pulmonary symptoms

- Work (job/school/play), community, and leisure integration or reintegration (including instrumental activities of daily living)

  Examples of examination findings include:
  - Ability to assume or resume work (job/school/plan), community, and leisure activities with or without assistive, adaptive, orthotic, protective, supportive, or prosthetic devices and equipment
  - Ability to gain access to work (job/school/play), community, and leisure environments
  - Safety in work (job/school/play), community, and leisure activities and environments

Evaluation

Evaluation is a thought process that may not include formal documentation.

However, the evaluation process may lead to documentation of impairments, activity limitations, and participation restrictions using formats such as:
- A problem list
- A statement of assessment of key factors (eg, cognitive factors, comorbidities, social support) influencing the patient/client status.

Diagnosis

Documentation of a diagnosis determined by the physical therapist may include impairment, activity limitation, and participation restrictions.

Examples include:
- Impaired Joint Mobility, Motor Function, Muscle Performance, and

  Range of Motion Associated With Localized Inflammation (4E)

- Impaired Motor Function and Sensory Integrity Associated With Progressive Disorders of the Central Nervous System (5E)
- Impaired Aerobic Capacity/Endurance Associated With Cardiovascular Pump Dysfunction or Failure (6D)
- Impaired Integumentary Integrity Associated With Partial-Thickness Skin Involvement and Scar Formation (7C)

Prognosis

Documentation of the prognosis is typically included in the plan of care. See below.

Plan of Care

Documentation of the plan of care includes the following:
- Overall goals stated in measurable terms that indicate the predicted level of improvement in functioning
- A general statement of interventions to be used
- Proposed duration and frequency of service required to reach the goals
- Anticipated discharge plans

VISIT/ENCOUNTER

Documentation of each visit/encounter shall include the following elements:
- Patient/client self-report (as appropriate).
- Identification of specific interventions provided, including frequency, intensity, and duration as appropriate. Examples include:
  - Knee extension, three sets, ten repetitions, 10# weight
  - Transfer training bed to chair with sliding board
  - Equipment provided
    - Changes in patient/client impairment, activity limitation, and participation restriction status as they relate to the plan of care.
    - Response to interventions, including adverse reactions, if any.
    - Factors that modify frequency or intensity of intervention and progression goals, including patient/client adherence to patient/client-related instructions.
    - Communication/consultation with providers/patient/client/family/ significant other.
    - Documentation to plan for ongoing provision of services for the next visit(s), which is suggested to include, but not be limited to:
      - The interventions with objectives
      - Progression parameters
      - Precautions, if indicated

REEXAMINATION

Documentation of reexamination shall include the following elements:
- Documentation of selected components of examination to update patient's/client's functioning, and/or disability status.
- Interpretation of findings and, when indicated, revision of goals.
- When indicated, revision of plan of care, as directly correlated with goals as documented.

DISCHARGE/DISCONTINUATION SUMMARY

Documentation of discharge or discontinuation shall include the following elements:

- Current physical/functional status.

- Degree of goals achieved and reasons for goals not being achieved.

- Discharge/discontinuation plan related to the patient/client's continuing care.

  Examples include:
  - Home program.
  - Referrals for additional services.
  - Recommendations for follow-up physical therapy care.
  - Family and caregiver training.
  - Equipment provided.

Relationship to Vision 2020: Professionalism
(Practice Department, ext 3176)
[Document updated: 12/14/2009]

Explanation of Reference Numbers:

BOD P00-00-00-00 stands for Board of Directors/month/year/page/vote in the Board of Directors Minutes; the "P" indicates that it is a position (see below). For example, BOD P11-97-06-18 means that this position can be found in the November 1997 Board of Directors minutes on Page 6 and that it was Vote 18.

P: Position | S: Standard | G: Guideline | Y: Policy | R: Procedure

Appendix B

Preferred Practice Patterns

MUSCULOSKELETAL

Pattern 4A: Primary Prevention/Risk Reduction for Skeletal Demineralization

Pattern 4B: Impaired Posture

Pattern 4C: Impaired Muscle Performance

Pattern 4D: Impaired Joint Mobility, Motor Function, Muscle Performance, and Range of Motion Associated With Connective Tissue Dysfunction

Pattern 4E: Impaired Joint Mobility, Motor Function, Muscle Performance, and Range of Motion Associated With Localized Inflammation

Pattern 4F: Impaired Joint Mobility, Motor Function, Muscle Performance, Range of Motion, and Reflex Integrity Associated With Spinal Disorders

Pattern 4G: Impaired Joint Mobility, Motor Function, Muscle Performance, and Range of Motion Associated With Fracture

Pattern 4H: Impaired Joint Mobility, Motor Function, Muscle Performance, and Range of Motion Associated With Joint Arthroplasty

Pattern 4I: Impaired Joint Mobility, Motor Function, Muscle Performance, and Range of Motion Associated With Bony or Soft Tissue Surgery

Pattern 4J: Impaired Joint Mobility, Motor Function, Muscle Performance, and Range of Motion, Gait, Locomotion, and Balance Associated With Amputation

NEUROMUSCULAR

Pattern 5A: Primary Prevention/Risk Reduction for Loss of Balance and Falling

Pattern 5B: Impaired Neuromotor Development

Pattern 5C: Impaired Motor Function and Sensory Integrity Associated With Nonprogressive Disorders of the Central Nervous System—Congenital Origin or Acquired in Infancy or Childhood

Pattern 5D: Impaired Motor Function and Sensory Integrity Associated With Nonprogressive Disorders of the Central Nervous System—Acquired in Adolescence of Adulthood

Pattern 5E: Impaired Motor Function and Sensory Integrity Associated With Progressive Disorders of the Central Nervous System

Erickson ML, Utzman RR, McKnight R. *Physical Therapy Documentation: From Examination to Outcome, Second Edition* (pp 147-148).
© 2014 SLACK Incorporated.

Pattern 5F: Impaired Peripheral Nerve Integrity and Muscle Performance Associated With Peripheral Nerve Injury

Pattern 5G: Impaired Motor Function and Sensory Integrity Associated With Acute or Chronic Polyneuropathies

Pattern 5H: Impaired Motor Function, Peripheral Nerve Integrity, and Sensory Integrity Associated With Nonprogressive Disorders of the Spinal Cord

Pattern 5I: Impaired Arousal, Range of Motion, and Motor Control Associated With Coma, Near Coma, or Vegetative State

CARDIOVASCULAR/PULMONARY

Pattern 6A: Primary Prevention/Risk Reduction for Cardiovascular/Pulmonary Disorders

Pattern 6B: Impaired Aerobic Capacity/Endurance Associated With Deconditioning

Pattern 6C: Impaired Ventilation, Respiration/Gas Exchange, and Aerobic Capacity/Endurance Associated With Airway Clearance Dysfunction

Pattern 6D: Impaired Aerobic Capacity/Endurance Associated With Cardiovascular Pump Dysfunction or Failure

Pattern 6E: Impaired Ventilation and Respiration/Gas Exchange Associated With Ventilatory Pump Dysfunction or Failure

Pattern 6F: Impaired Ventilation and Respiration/Gas Exchange Associated With Respiratory Failure

Pattern 6G: Impaired Ventilation, Respiration/Gas Exchange, and Aerobic Capacity/Endurance Associated With Respiratory Failure in the Neonate

Pattern 6H: Impaired Circulation and Anthropometric Dimensions Associated With Lymphatic System Disorders

INTEGUMENTARY

Pattern 7A: Primary Prevention/Risk Reduction for Integumentary Disorders

Pattern 7B: Impaired Integumentary Integrity Associated With Superficial Skin Involvement

Pattern 7C: Impaired Integumentary Integrity Associated With Partial-Thickness Skin Involvement and Scar Formation

Pattern 7D: Impaired Integumentary Integrity Associated With Full-Thickness Involvement and Scar Formation

Pattern 7E: Impaired Integumentary Integrity Associated With Skin Involvement Extending Into Fascia, Muscle, or Bone and Scar Formation

Sample Forms

Erickson ML, Utzman RR, McKnight R. *Physical Therapy Documentation:*
From Examination to Outcome, Second Edition (pp 149-155).
© 2014 SLACK Incorporated.

PHYSICAL THERAPY EXAMINATION

Patient's Name _____ Age _____ Date of Examination _____

Referred by: _____ for: _____

Medical Diagnosis _____ DOI/Onset _____

Affected side: ☐ Right   ☐ Left   ☐ Both   Hand Dominance: ☐ Right   ☐ Left

Gender: ☐ Male   ☐ Female

History:

History of Present Illness (HPI): _____

_____

_____

Chief complaint: _____

History of similar problem: ☐ No   ☐ Yes, describe: _____

PMH/Comorbidities/Complexities: ☐ None   ☐ Yes _____

_____

Surgical history: ☐ None   ☐ Yes _____

Significant family history: ☐ None   ☐ Yes _____

Current services being received for this problem: ☐ None   ☐ Yes _____

Prior treatment for this problem (including PT): ☐ None   ☐ Yes _____

Medications: ☐ None   ☐ Yes _____

Drug allergies: ☐ None   ☐ Yes _____

Imaging studies for present problem: ☐ None   ☐ Yes _____

Orthotic/assistive/prosthetic devices: ☐ None   ☐ Yes _____

For chronic conditions: Recent change in status: _____

Date of change/decline: _____ New safety issues: _____

Functional level before change: _____

_____

Living Environment/Situation: _____

Available social support: _____

Requires Assistance: ☐ No   ☐ Yes _____

Obstacles: ☐ No   ☐ Yes _____

General health/health habits: _____

    ☐ See attached general health questionnaire

Current/Prior Functional Status:

    ADL: _____

    Home management tasks: _____

    Community tasks: _____

    Occupation/Work status/School: _____

      Requirements:_____

    Recreation/Leisure: _____

    Global Rating (0-100%): _____

    ☐ See attached self-report disability/functional questionnaire

Patient's Therapy Goals: _____

Need for PT: ☐ Return to PLOF   ☐ Decrease assistance currently required
            ☐ Change in living environment

Patient concerns: _____

Pain: Verbal rating (0-10): _____

Description: _____

Frequency/Duration of Pain: _____

Activities that: increase pain: _____   decrease pain: _____

Numbness/Tingling: ☐ None   ☐ Yes, Location: _____

Temperature changes: ☐ None   ☐ Yes, Location: _____

Gross Review of Systems:

Cardiopulmonary: BP _____ HR _____ RR _____ O$_2$ sat _____

                         ☐ Not impaired   ☐ Impaired _____

                         ☐ (see specific exam below)

Integumentary: ☐ Not impaired   ☐ Impaired _____

                         ☐ (see specific exam below)

Musculoskeletal: ☐ Not impaired   ☐ Impaired _____

                         ☐ (see specific exam below)

Neurological: ☐ Not impaired   ☐ Impaired _____

                         ☐ (see specific exam below)

Cognitive/Communicative Ability: ☐ Not impaired   ☐ Impaired _____

Physical Therapy Tests/Measures:
(identify/list those done frequently)

(include impairments and function)

(include space for "Other")

Functional assessment(s): ☐ See attached functional assessment (Berg Balance Test, FIM, etc)

Today's Interventions:

Collaboration/Communication: ☐ None   ☐ Yes _____

HEP Instructions: _____
_____
_____

Other Pt. Education: _____
_____
_____

     Pt./caregiver response to teaching: _____
_____

Procedural Interventions: _____
_____
_____
_____

PHYSICAL THERAPY ASSESSMENT AND PLAN (PLAN OF CARE)

Patient Name: _____ Patient's DOB: _____ PT Examination Date _____

★★ For the physician:
I have read and concur with the plan of care written below for this patient:

_____   _____   _____
Name of Supervising Physician   Physician Signature   Date

Summary/Comments: _____
_____
Primary Medical Diagnosis: (ICD-9) _____
PT Diagnosis: _____
Factors influencing treatment : _____
Patient's Rehab Potential: _____

Problem List:

Physical therapy impairments:	*Activity Limitations and Participation Restrictions:* *(Include ADL, home management, community, work, leisure)*
1.	1.
2.	2.
3.	3.
4.	4.
5.	5.

Expected Outcomes (to be met by _____):
      A.
      B.
      C.
      D.
      E.
STGs (to be met by _____):
      A-1.
      B-1.
      C-1.
      D-1.
      E-1.

Medicare G Code _____   Severity _____   Goal _____

Treatment Plan:
Skilled services will be provided for: _____
_____
Frequency/Duration services will be provided: _____
☐ The patient/caregiver is in agreement with the plan.
Examination, assessment, and plan of care completed and written by: _____
                                                 (PT Signature)

Physical therapy modality/procedure code(s)	
1.	4.
2.	5.
3.	6.

REFERENCES

1. American Physical Therapy Association. *Guidelines: Physical Therapy Documentation of Patient/Client Management* BOD G03-05-16-41. http://www.apta.org/uploadedFiles/APTAorg/About_Us/Policies/BOD/Practice/DocumentationPatientClient Mgmt.pdf. Accessed May 16, 2012.
2. American Physical Therapy Association. *Guide to Physical Therapist Practice*. 2nd ed. Alexandria, VA: APTA; 2003.
3. Centers for Medicare and Medicaid Services. Covered medical and other health services. *Medicare Benefit Policy Manual*. Publication 100-02. http://www.cms.gov/Regulations-and-Guidance/Guidance/Manuals/Downloads/bp102c15.pdf. Accessed May 16, 2012.

Treatment Encounter Note #_____

Patient Name _____   Date _____

Subjective Report _____
_____
_____
_____

Objective Measurements _____
_____
_____
_____
_____
_____

Interventions (communication, education, and procedural interventions):

_____ Total timed code minutes   _____ Total treatment time

Response to treatment _____
_____
_____

Change(s) in status since initial visit _____
_____
_____

Factors warranting change to plan of care _____
_____
_____

Plans for next visit _____
_____

Signature(s)_____

PROGRESS REPORT

Patient Name _____   Dates of service _____

Date Progress Report written _____

Subjective Report _____

_____

_____

_____

Objective Measurements _____

_____

_____

_____

Current Outcome Goals to be met by _____	Progress toward goals:
A.	
B.	
C.	
D.	
E.	
F.	

Medicare G Code _____   Severity: Initial _____   Current _____   Goal _____

Interventions (Include treatment time and total time): _____

_____

_____

Changes to plan of care and rationale: _____

_____

_____

_____

Plans for further interventions: _____

_____

_____

_____

★★ **For the physician:**

I have read and concur with the plan of care for this patient:

_____   _____   _____

Name of Supervising Physician   Physician Signature   Date

Abbreviations and Symbols

This list provides many of the abbreviations and symbols used in medical charts and in physical therapy records. Because documentation styles can vary, you should check with your facility regarding abbreviations and symbols that are "approved" for use. Also, note that some abbreviations have more than one meaning. Be careful and understand the context in which each abbreviation is used.

ABBREVIATIONS

A

(A), (a) or ⓐ	assist
A: or A	assessment
AAROM	active assistive range of motion
Ab	antibody
abd	abduction
ABG(s)	arterial blood gas(es)
ABN	advanced beneficiary notice
ac	before meals
ACE	angiotensin-converting enzyme
Ach	acetylcholine
ACL	anterior cruciate ligament
ACO	accountable care organization
AD	assistive device; Alzheimer's disease
ADA	Americans with Disabilities Act
add	adduction
ADL	activities of daily living
ad lib	as desired
ADM	abductor digiti minimi
AE	above elbow
AFB	acid-fast bacilli
AFO	ankle-foot orthosis
AGA	appropriate for gestational age
AIDS	acquired immunodeficiency syndrome

AK	above knee
AKA	above knee amputation
ALL	acute lymphoblastic leukemia
ALS	amyotrophic lateral sclerosis
am	before noon
AMA	against medical advice; American Medical Association
AMB	ambulatory
AML	acute myeloblastic leukemia
AMP	Amputee Mobility Predictor
ANOVA	analysis of variance
AP	ankle pump; anterior-posterior
APB	abductor pollicis brevis
APL	abductor pollicis longus
APTA	American Physical Therapy Association
ARDS	adult (acute) respiratory distress syndrome
AROM	active range of motion
ARRA	American Recovery and Reinvestment Act
ASA	aspirin
ASAP	as soon as possible
ASHD	arteriosclerotic heart disease
ATF	anterior talofibular
AV	atriovenous

Erickson ML, Utzman RR, McKnight R. *Physical Therapy Documentation: From Examination to Outcome, Second Edition* (pp 157-162). © 2014 SLACK Incorporated.

B

Ba	barium
BBB	blood-brain barrier
BE	below elbow
BI	brain injury
bid	twice daily
BK	below knee
BKA	below knee amputation
BLE or (B)LE	bilateral lower extremities
BM	bowel movement
BMD	bone mineral density
BMI	body mass index
BP	blood pressure
BPH	benign prostatic hypertrophy
BPM or bpm	beats per minute
BRP	bathroom privileges
BSA	body surface area
BUE or (B)UE	bilateral upper extremities
BUN	blood urea nitrogen

C

Ca	calcium
CA	cancer
CABG	coronary artery bypass graft
CAD	coronary artery disease
CAT	computerized axial tomography
CBC	complete blood count
c/c or C/C	chief complaint
cc or cm³	cubic centimeter
CCU	critical (or coronary) care unit
CDC	Centers for Disease Control and Prevention
C. diff	*Clostridium difficile*
CDO	care delivery organization
CF	calcaneofibular; cystic fibrosis
CGA	contact guard assist
CHI	closed head injury
CHO	carbohydrate
Cl	chlorine
cm	centimeter
CMC	carpometacarpal
CMS	Centers for Medicare & Medicaid Services
CMV	cytomegalovirus
CNS	central nervous system
c/o or C/O	complains of
COPD	chronic obstructive pulmonary disease
CORF	comprehensive outpatient rehabilitation facility
COTA	certified occupational therapist assistant
CP	cerebral palsy
CPAP	continuous positive airway pressure
CPM	continuous passive motion
CPT	Common Procedural Terminology
CRNP	Certified Registered Nurse Practitioner
CPR	cardiopulmonary resuscitation
C & S	culture and sensitivity

CSF	cerebrospinal fluid
CT	computed tomography
CV	cardiovascular
CVA	cerebrovascular accident
CWP	cold whirlpool
cx	cancel; crutches

D

DASH	Disabilities of the Arm, Shoulder, and Hand (outcomes measure)
DBS	deep brain stimulator (stimulation)
d/c	discharge; discontinue
DC	doctor of chiropractic; chiropractor
DD	developmental delay
DDD	degenerative disc disease
dep.	dependent
dept.	department
DF	dorsiflexion
DHHR	Department of Health and Human Resources
DI	dorsal interossei
DIP	distal interphalangeal
DJD	degenerative joint disease
DM	diabetes mellitus
DME	durable medical equipment
DMERC	durable medical equipment regional carrier
DNR	do not resuscitate
DO	doctor of osteopath
DOI	date of injury
DRG	diagnosis-related group
DRUJ	distal radioulnar joint
DTR	deep tendon reflex
DVT	deep vein thrombosis
dx	diagnosis

E

ea.	each
EBP	evidence-based practice
ECF	extracellular fluid
E. coli	*Escherichia coli*
ECRB	extensor carpi radialis brevis
ECRL	extensor carpi radialis longus
ECU	extensor carpi ulnaris
ED	emergency department
EDC	extensor digitorum communis
EDM	extensor digiti minimi
EEG	electroencephalogram
EENT	eyes, ears, nose, and throat
EHR	electronic health record
EIP	extensor indicis proprius
EKG, ECG	electrocardiogram
EMG	electromyogram
EMR	electronic medical record
EMS	emergency medical services
ENG	electronystagmograph
EO	elbow orthosis
EOB	explanation of benefits

EPB	extensor pollicis brevis
EPL	extensor pollicis longus
ER	external rotation; emergency room
ERV	expiratory reserve volume
ES	effect size
ESR	erythrocyte sedimentation rate
ESRD	end-stage renal disease
ET	endotracheal
EtOH or ETOH	ethyl alcohol
ev or ever	eversion
eval.	evaluation
ex.	exercise

F

F or 3/5	fair (manual muscle test)
FBS	fasting blood sugar
FCE	functional capacity evaluation
FCR	flexor carpi radialis
FCU	flexor carpi ulnaris
FDA	US Food and Drug Administration
FDM	flexor digiti minimi
FDP	flexor digitorum profundus
FDS	flexor digitorum superficialis
FES	functional electrical stimulation
FEV	forced expiratory volume
FHR	fetal heart rate
FIM	Functional Independence Measure
fl	fluid
FM or FMS	fibromyalgia syndrome
FO	foot orthosis
FOR	functional outcome report
FPB	flexor pollicis brevis
FPL	flexor pollicis longus
FRC	functional residual capacity
FSBPT	Federation of State Boards of Physical Therapy
FTSG	full-thickness skin graft
FU or F/U	follow-up
FUO	fever of unknown origin
FVC	forced vital capacity
FWB	full weight bearing
FWW	front-wheeled walker
fx	fracture

G

G or 4/5	good (manual muscle test)
g	gram
GA	gestational age
GERD	gastroesophageal reflux disease
GH	glenohumeral
GI	gastrointestinal
GS	gluteal sets
GTT	glucose tolerance test

H

H_2O	water
h, hr, or hr.	hour
HAV	hepatitis A virus; hallux abductovalgus

Hb	hemoglobin
HBV	hepatitis B virus
HCFA	Health Care Financing Administration
HCPCS	health care common procedure coding system
Hct	hematocrit
HCV	hepatitis C virus
HDL	high-density lipoprotein
HEP	home exercise program
H & H	hemoglobin and hematocrit
HHA	home health agency
HIT	health information technology
HITECH	Health Information Technology for Economic and Clinical Health Act
HIV	human immunodeficiency virus
HMO	health maintenance organization
HNP	herniated nucleus pulposus
h/o	history of
HO	hand orthosis; hip orthosis
HOB	head of bed
H & P	history and physical
HP	hot pack
HPI	history of present illness
HR	handrail; heart rate
HRT	hormone replacement therapy
HTN	hypertension
hx	history
Hz	hertz

I

I or (I)	independent
IADL	instrumental activities of daily living
IC	inspiratory capacity
ICD	International Classification of Disease
ICF	intracellular fluid; International Classification of Functioning, Disability, and Health
ICIDH	International Classification of Impairments, Disabilities, and Handicaps
ICHI	International Classification of Health Interventions
ICP	intracranial pressure
ICU	intensive care unit
I & D	incision and drainage
IDDM	insulin-dependent diabetes mellitus
IDEA	Individuals with Disabilities in Education Act
IEP	Individualized Education Plan
IFSP	Individualized Family Service Plan
Ig	immunoglobulin
IM	intramuscular
INH	isoniazid
inv	inversion
I & O	intake and output
IP	inpatient; interphalangeal
IPPS	inpatient prospective payment system
IR	internal rotation

IRF	Inpatient Rehabilitation Facility	MS	multiple sclerosis
IRFPAI	Inpatient Rehabilitation Facility Patient Assessment Instrument	MTP	metatarsophalangeal
		mV	millivolt
IRV	inspiratory reserve volume	μV	microvolt
IV	intravenous		

N

		N or 5/5	normal (manual muscle test)
K		N	newton
K	potassium	n.	nerve
KAFO	knee-ankle-foot orthosis	Na	sodium
kg	kilogram	N/A	not applicable
KO	knee orthosis	NBQC	narrow base quad cane
		NCMRR	National Center for Medical Rehabilitation Research

L

Ⓛ, L, or (L)	left	NDI	Neck Disability Index
L	liter	NDT	neurodevelopmental treatment
LAC	long arm cast	NICU	neonatal intensive care unit
LAQ	long arc quadriceps exercise	NIDDM	noninsulin-dependent diabetes mellitus
LCL	lateral collateral ligament	NIH	National Institutes of Health
LDL	low-density lipoprotein	NMES	neuromuscular electrical stimulation
LE	lower extremity	NPO	nothing by mouth
LHD	left hand dominant	n.s.	at bedtime
LLC	long leg cast	NSAID(s)	nonsteroidal anti-inflammatory drug(s)
LMN	lower motor neuron	NT	not tested
LMRP	local medical review policies	n & v	nausea and vomiting
LP	lumbar puncture	NWB	nonweight bearing
L/S, l/s	lifestyle		
LT	lunotriquetral	**O**	
LTFG	long-term functional goal	O: or O	objective
LTG	long-term goal	O2 or O_2	oxygen
LTM	long-term memory	OA	osteoarthritis
		OASIS	outcome and assessment information set

M

m	meter	OB/GYN	obstetrics and gynecology
m.	muscle	OBS	organic brain syndrome
max	maximum	OCD	obsessive compulsive disorder
MCID	minimal clinically important difference	ODM	opponens digiti minimi
		OI	osteogenesis imperfecta
MCL	medial collateral ligament	OOB	out of bed
MCP	metacarpophalangeal	OP	opponens pollicis; outpatient
MD	muscular dystrophy; medical doctor/physician	OR	operating room
		ORIF	open reduction internal fixation
MDC	minimal detectable charge	OSHA	Occupational Safety & Health Administration
MDS	minimum data set		
MED(S) or meds	medicines, medications	OT	occupational therapist
MG	myasthenia gravis	OTC	over-the-counter (ie, drugs)
MHz	megahertz	OTR/L	occupational therapist registered and licensed
MI	myocardial infarction		
MID	multi-infarct dementia	oz or oz.	ounce
min	minimal		
mm	millimeter	**P**	
mm Hg	millimeters of mercury	P or 2/5	poor (manual muscle test)
MMT	manual muscle test	P: or P	plan
mod	moderate	p!	pain
MOI	mechanism of injury	PA	posteroanterior
mos	months	PA-C	physician assistant
MRI	magnetic resonance image	pc	after meals
MRSA	methicillin-resistant *Staphylococcus aureus*	PCA	patient-controlled anesthesia
		PCL	posterior cruciate ligament

PD	Parkinson disease		RBC	red blood cell
PDR	*Physicians' Desk Reference*		RC	radiocarpal
PE	pulmonary embolism		RCL	radial collateral ligament
PEG	percutaneous endoscopic gastrostomy (tube)		RD	radial deviation
			RDS	respiratory distress syndrome
PERRLA	pupils equal, round (regular), reactive to light, and accommodating		reps	repetitions
			RGO	reciprocating gait orthosis
PET	positron emission tomography		RHD	right hand dominant
PF	plantarflexion		R/O or r/o	rule out
PFT	pulmonary function test		ROM	range of motion
PHI	protected health information		RPE	rate of perceived exertion
PI	palmar interossei		RR	respiratory rate
PIP	proximal interphalangeal		R/S or r/s	reschedule
PL	palmaris longus		RT	respiratory therapy
PLOF	prior level of function		RTC	return to clinic
pm	after noon		RTW	return to work
PMH	past (prior, previous) medical history		RUG	resource utilization group
PNF	proprioceptive neuromuscular facilitation		RV	residual volume
PNS	peripheral nervous system		RVU	relative value units
po	by mouth		Rx	prescription
POMR	problem-oriented medical record			
post-op	postoperative		**S**	
PPO	preferred provider organization		S: or S	subjective
PPS	prospective payment system		SAC	short arm cast
PQ	pronator quadratus		SaO$_2$	oxygen saturation
Pr:	problem		SAQ	short arc quadriceps exercise
PRN	as needed		SBA	stand by assist
PROM	passive range of motion		SCI	spinal cord injury
PRUJ	proximal radioulnar joint		SEWHFO	shoulder-elbow-wrist-hand-finger orthosis
PT	physical therapist; pronator teres; prothrombin time		SF-36	Short-Form Health Survey
Pt. or pt.	patient		SIDS	sudden infant death syndrome
PTA	physical therapist assistant; prior to admission		SL	scapholunate; side lying
			SLC	short leg cast
PTCA	percutaneous transluminal coronary angioplasty		SLE	systemic lupus erythematosus
			SLP	speech language pathologist
PTF	posterior talofibular		SLR	straight leg raise
PTT	partial thromboplastin time		SMA	spinal muscular atrophy
PVD	peripheral vascular disease		SNF	skilled nursing facility
PWB	partial weight bearing (usually 50% unless otherwise indicated; may need to check with physician to clarify)		SO	shoulder orthosis
			SOB	shortness of breath
			s/p	status post
			SPT	student physical therapist
Q			SPTA	student physical therapist assistant
q	every		s/s	signs and symptoms
q2h	every 2 hours		ST	scapulothoracic
q3h	every 3 hours		stat	immediately
q4h	every 4 hours		STG	short-term goal
q8h	every 8 hours		STM	short-term memory
qam	every morning		SVN or s	supervision
qh	every hour		STSG	split-thickness skin graft
qid	four times a day			
qod	every other day		**T**	
QS or qs	quad set/quadriceps set			
			T or 1/5	trace (manual muscle test)
R			T	temperature
Ⓡ or (R)	right		TA	therapeutic activity
			TB	tuberculosis
RA	rheumatoid arthritis		TBI	traumatic brain injury

T or tbsp	tablespoon
TDWB	touch-down weight bearing
TENS	transcutaneous electrical nerve stimulation
TFCC	triangular fibrocartilaginous complex
THA	total hip arthroplasty
THR	total hip replacement
TIA	transient ischemic attack
tid	three times a day
TJC	The Joint Commission
TKA	total knee arthroplasty
TKE	terminal knee extension
TKR	total knee replacement
TMJ	temporomandibular joint
TP	therapeutic procedure
TPN	total parenteral nutrition
t or tsp	teaspoon
TTP	tender to palpation
TTWB	toe touch weight bearing
TUG	Timed Up and Go
TV	tidal volume
tx	traction or treatment

U

UCL	ulnar collateral ligament
UD	ulnar deviation
UE	upper extremity
UMN	upper motor neuron

US	ultrasound
UTI	urinary tract infection
UV	ultraviolet

V

V	volt

W

W	watt
WBAT	weight bearing as tolerated
WBC	white blood cell
WBQC	wide base quad cane
w/c	wheelchair
w/cm²	watts per centimeters squared
WFL	within functional limits
WHFO	wrist-hand-finger orthosis
WHO	wrist-hand orthosis; World Health Organization
WHOFIC	World Health Organization Family of International Classifications
wk	week
WNL	within normal limits
WP	whirlpool
WWP	warm whirlpool

Y

y.o. or yo	year old

COMMON SYMBOLS

about	~
after	$\bar{p}$
ascend or increase	↑
assist (min, mod, max assist)	ⓐ, (a), or (A)
at	@
before	$\bar{a}$
both or bilateral	bil., B, (B), or Ⓑ
degrees	°
degrees Celsius	°C
degrees Fahrenheit	°F
dependent	(D) or dep.
descend or decrease	↓
equal, equal to	(=)
extension	/
female	♀
flexion	✓
from	←
greater than, greater than or equal to	>, ≥
hour, foot	'
inch, minute	"
independent	(I), or Ⓘ
left	Ⓛ, (L), or L

less than, less than or equal to	<, ≤
male	♂
micron	µ
negative	(–) or –
not equal to, unequal	≠
number of individuals assisting (one, two)	×1, ×2
parallel (as in parallel bars)	// (// bars)
per	/
positive	(+) or +
possible, question, suggestive	?
pounds	# or lbs.
primary	1°
right	Ⓡ, (R), or R
sample mean	$\bar{x}$
secondary, secondary to	2°, 2° to
times (as in 3 times per day)	× (eg, 3×/day)
to	→
to and from	↔
up and down or ascend and descend	↑↓
with	$\bar{c}$
without	$\bar{s}$

Assessing Change

Many authors are currently reporting the standard error of the measurement (SEM), minimal detectable change (MDC), and/or minimal clinically imperfect difference (MCID) associated with clinical tests and measures. However, this has not always been the case and these values are not known for many instruments we use clinically. Therefore, the following formulas are provided so that values can be extrapolated from more general literature.[1]
The SEM is calculated in the following manner[1]:

$$SEM = \text{standard deviation} \times \sqrt{(1 - \text{reliability coefficient})}$$

When estimating the SEM for a questionnaire with multiple items, administered at a single point in time (or for a one-time use), the reliability coefficient used is the Cronbach's α value[2]:

$$SEM = \text{standard deviation} \times \sqrt{(1 - \text{Cronbach's } \alpha)}$$

However, when estimating the SEM for a change score, the test-retest reliability coefficient (ICC) is used to calculate the SEM[1,3]:

$$SEM_{\text{test-retest}} = \text{standard deviation}_{\text{baseline}} \times \sqrt{(1 - ICC)}$$

The MDC (with a 95% confidence interval) is calculated using the SEM in the following manner[1]:

$$MDC_{95} = SEM_{\text{test-retest}} \times \text{z-value}_{95} \times \sqrt{2}$$
$$or: \quad MDC_{95} = SEM_{\text{test-retest}} \times 1.96 \times \sqrt{2}$$

Erickson ML, Utzman RR, McKnight R. *Physical Therapy Documentation: From Examination to Outcome, Second Edition* (pp 163-164).
© 2014 SLACK Incorporated.

Authors examining psychometric properties of the disabilities of the arm, shoulder, and hand (DASH) used this formula to calculate the MDC of the DASH (MDC_{95}).[3] First, they calculated the test-retest SEM ($SEM_{test-retest}$) at the 95% confidence level using the ICC value (.96) and the baseline standard deviation (23.02) (see box below). Second, they calculated the SEM at the 95% confidence level (SEM_{95}) as described above. Then, they multiplied the SEM_{95} by the square root of two to determine the MDC_{95}[3]:

Step One:

$SEM_{test-retest} = \text{standard deviation}_{baseline} \times \sqrt{(1\text{-ICC})}$

$SEM_{test-retest} = (23.02 \times \sqrt{1\text{-}.96})$

$SEM_{test-retest} = 4.6$ DASH points

Step Two:

$SEM_{95} = SEM \times z\text{-value}_{95}$

$SEM_{95} = 4.6 \times 1.96$

$SEM_{95} = 9$ DASH points

Step Three:

$MDC_{95} = SEM_{95} \times \sqrt{2}$

$MDC_{95} = 9 \times \sqrt{2}$

$MDC_{95} = 12.75$ DASH points

REFERENCES

1. MacDermid JC, Stratford P. Applying evidence on outcome measures to hand therapy practice. *J Hand Ther*. 2004;17:165-173.
2. Michener LA, Leggin BG. A review of self-report scales for the assessment of hand function. *J Hand Ther*. 2001;14:68-76.
3. Beaton DE, Katz JN, Fossel AH, Wright JG, Tarasuk V. Measuring the whole or parts: validity, reliability, and responsiveness of the DASH outcome measure in different regions of the upper extremity. *J Hand Ther*. 2001;14:128-146.

Glossary

abuse: Billing for items that are not covered or misusing billing codes. Usually a result of an error or unawareness of the proper code(s) or coding procedure(s).

activities of daily living (ADL): Skills required to be independent in day-to-day living (ie, bathing, grooming, self-care, mobility, toileting, transfers).

activity: Completion of a task or action by an individual.

activity limitation: Difficulties or limitations encountered by an individual who is attempting to complete a task or carry out an activity.

addendum: An entry made into the medical record that "adds" new information to an already existing note that is completed and signed; follows the original documentation without skipping lines and is titled, "Addendum:."

advance beneficiary notice (ABN): A notification that a health care provider asks a Medicare beneficiary to sign when providing a service that is not or may not be covered by Medicare. In signing the ABN, the Medicare beneficiary agrees to pay for the service if it is not covered by Medicare.

assessment: The physical therapist's clinical judgment or overall impression of the patient. The A: section of a SOAP. In the SOAP note, includes a brief patient summary, rehab potential, medical and/or PT diagnosis, expected goals and potential for achievement; may also include patient progress or regression, status toward existing goals, overall improvement, or justification/need for skilled services.

attribute: A variable; a characteristic or quality that is measured.

auditor: A person who checks accounts of an individual, group, or organization. An auditor for an insurance company may review a provider's records to determine if services that were provided to a patient are consistent with what was billed.

authenticate: A process that verifies a note is complete, genuine, and accurate; usually done in the form of applying the signature of the individual writing the note.

capacity: Extent of an activity limitation; direct manifestations of the health state including activities performed without assistance; scored in Activities and Participation Domain for ICF evaluation scheme.

carrier: A privately run insurance company that contracts with the government to pay bills for Medicare Part B. Carriers are determined by geographic region and can be found at http://www.cms.hhs.gov/contacts/incardir. asp#4.

case-mix group: Categorization or grouping of patients who are admitted to hospitals, or other facilities, according to common characteristics such diagnosis, disease, and functional status.

Centers for Medicare & Medicaid Services (CMS): A federal government agency that administers Medicare and works with state governments to administer Medicaid and State Children's Health Insurance Programs (SCHIP). CMS is housed within the Department of Health and Human Services (www.cms.hhs.gov).

claim: The process of submitting a bill to an insurance company; may be made by the patient or the health care provider, depending on the insurance plan.

coding: The process of assigning codes to describe a patient's health care problem and/or the services rendered.

cohort: A group of people with similar characteristics.

common procedural terminology (CPT): A system for coding procedures provided to patients. The CPT coding system is developed by the American Medical Association, which regularly updates the codes to reflect current practice.

comorbidity (*or* comorbidities): Aspect(s) of the patient's past medical history that affect(s) his or her current episode of care; or a previous or current medical condition that has the potential to hinder or slow progress in physical therapy.

compliance: The ongoing process of keeping current on laws, regulations, and policies impacting the delivery and payment for health care services and practicing within those laws, regulations, and policies.

contextual factors: Factors, usually facilitators or barriers, that are either internal or external to an individual that influence his or her ability to participate in society.

copayment: Many health insurance plans require a patient to pay a portion of the cost of services provided; this portion is referred to a copayment. For example, a patient is covered by a health insurance plan that requires the patient pay a $20 copayment for each physical therapy visit. For each visit, the patient pays $20; the insurance plan pays the remainder of the charge for the visit.

Erickson ML, Utzman RR, McKnight R. *Physical Therapy Documentation: From Examination to Outcome, Second Edition* (pp 165-170).
© 2014 SLACK Incorporated.

core set: A specific set of items from the ICF that are specific to a given disease, injury, or condition.

Cronbach's alpha (α): A reliability value given as a measure of internal consistency.

deductible: A term used to refer to the amount a patient must pay before his or her insurance will take over payment. For instance, if a patient is covered by an insurance plan with a $500 deductible, the patient is responsible for paying the first $500 of care provided during a year. After reaching the $500 deductible, the patient's insurance plan will begin paying for covered health care services.

diagnosis (Dx): A medical diagnosis, assigned by the physician, identifies the injury, illness, or disease, usually at the cellular, organ, or system level. A physical therapy diagnosis, assigned by the physical therapist, identifies the impact of the patient's medical diagnosis and impairments on movement and function.

diagnosis-related group (DRG): A categorization system used to group patients according to diagnosis, type of treatment, age, and other relevant criteria. DRGs are used as part of the inpatient prospective payment system.

dictation: Providing verbal communication that is later transcribed (copied into written text).

disability: The inability or limitation in performing socially defined roles and/or tasks that would normally be expected of an individual within a given culture and/or environment.

disablement: The consequences of disease as they pertain to the relationship between body structures, ability to carry out tasks, and ability to function within society.

disablement framework (model): Conceptual framework used to describe disability in terms of disease/injury, impairments on body systems, and ability to carry out meaningful life tasks.

discharge (D/C): Terminating care provided to a patient at the end of an episode of care when expected goals have been achieved.

discharge goal: The intended result of patient/client management; the anticipated or expected changes in impairment, activity limitation, or participation restrictions and the time frame required to achieve.

discharge summary: Part of the physical therapy documentation. Written at the end of an episode of care, when the patient is discharged from a facility or provider or when physical therapy services are discontinued. Summarizes the care provided, patient progress, and final outcome.

discontinuation: A process described in the *Guide to Physical Therapist Practice* as the termination of services during a single episode of care when a (1) patient/family member/caregiver declines or refuses further interventions; (2) patient cannot meet the expected goals because of medical, psychosocial, or financial reasons; or (3) physical therapist feels the patient will no longer benefit.

documentation: A record of any aspect of patient/client management.

durable medical equipment (DME): Medical equipment that has been prescribed by a health care provider that is either purchased or rented by a patient to be used in the patient's home. Examples include hospital beds, walkers, canes, wheelchairs, and oxygen.

electronic health record (EHR): A record of all the health care an individual receives across the life span in a variety of delivery organizations; owned by the patient.

electronic medical record (EMR): A record of a patient's care provided in a single care delivery organization; owned by the care delivery organization.

environmental factors: External factors, immediate or global, that affect the individual as he or she interacts with society; can be physical, social, or attitudinal barriers, adaptations, or accommodations.

episode of (physical therapy) care: All physical therapy services that are (1) provided by a physical therapist, (2) provided in an unbroken sequence, and (3) related to the problem or related to a request from the patient/client, family, or other health care provider. The episode of care may include transfers between sites within or across settings or reclassification of the patient/client from one preferred practice pattern to another.

evaluation: An assessment of the patient's condition based on data collected during the examination that is performed by the physical therapist. It includes consideration of the chronicity, severity, complexity, and extent of impairments, functional limitations, and disabilities.

evidence-based practice (EBP): Using the best evidence available (research reports, case studies, textbooks, etc) along with clinical experience to make patient care decisions.

examination: A collection of tests and measurements, including questions to determine previous medical history, complaints, lifestyle, and physical therapy goals. The examination data are used to identify pertinent physical therapy problems, comorbidities, and rehabilitation potential; to determine expected outcomes; and to develop a plan of care that includes appropriate interventions, consultation with other health care providers, and patient education.

expected outcome: *See* discharge goal.

fiscal intermediary (*also known as* Intermediary): A privately run insurance company that contracts with the government to pay bills for Medicare Part A and some Part B. Fiscal intermediaries are determined by geographic region and can be found at http://www.cms.hhs.gov/contacts/incardir.asp#4.

fraud: Billing an insurance company, Medicare, or other third-party payer for services that were not provided, or billing for an item or service that has higher reimbursement than the service or item provided.

functional assessment: A patient assessment performed by a health care provider designed to measure a patient's functional capacity or capability.

functional independence measure (FIM): A standardized, multidisciplinary evaluation tool often used to score the patient's performance in self-care, bowel and bladder management, transfers, gait and/or wheelchair mobility, communication, and cognition. Patients are scored 1 to 7 (1 equal to total assist and 7 equal to independent) according to the level of assist they require to complete the task.

functional limitation: An abnormality or limitation in an individual's ability to carry out a meaningful action, task, and/or activity that is the result of a pathology and/or impairment(s).

functional outcome report (FOR): A format for documentation that focuses on the ability to perform meaningful functional activities rather than isolated musculoskeletal, neuromuscular, cardiopulmonary, or integumentary impairments.

health information clearinghouse: An entity associated with a health care provider or third-party payer that provides services such as billing, database management, transcription, or information technology. The health care clearinghouse has access to patient information but is not involved in patient care.

Health Insurance Portability and Accountability Act (HIPAA): A federal law enacted in 1996. The law includes provisions for workers to maintain health insurance coverage when they change jobs, to safeguard privacy of patient's confidential health information, and to combat health care fraud.

history taking: Gathering of data from the present and the past related to why the patient is seeking physical therapy services. The data are collected through patient/family interview and medical history review.

home health care: Skilled nursing or rehabilitative care provided in a patient's home. Home care services can be provided when a patient is declared "homebound."

homebound: Status given to a patient when he or she is unable to leave his or her home, or when leaving requires significantly taxing efforts. Short, infrequent trips, such as medical appointments and religious services, are permitted when a patient has been declared "homebound."

impairment: A deviation or loss in a body function or structure.

incident report: A report filed in the event of an "incident" that could likely result in a lawsuit. Used to document errors and departures from normal procedures that result in adverse outcomes, procedural breakdowns, and catastrophic events. These reports are filed by the individual involved in the incident and filed with the risk management department.

informed consent: Consent to a treatment(s) or service(s) given by a patient after being informed of risks, benefits, alternatives, and consequences of no treatment at all.

inpatient rehabilitation facility (IRF): A hospital, or unit within a larger facility (ie, acute care hospital), that provides intense rehabilitative services to patients. The majority of patients admitted to an IRF have been diagnosed with 1 of 13 qualifying medical conditions that have been established by Medicare. Examples are stroke, spinal cord injury, brain injury, amputation, hip fracture, burn, neurological disorder, and knee or hip replacement. More information and the list of qualifying diagnoses can be found at http://www.cms.hhs.gov/medlearn/matters/mmarticles/2004/MM3334.pdf.

interim note: Part of the physical therapy documentation; notes reflecting care provided after the initial examination and evaluation.

International Classification of Disease (ICD): A system of classifying patient illnesses and injuries by diagnosis. The 10th edition, ICD-10, is the most current version. The 9th edition, ICD-9, is still used commonly for insurance reimbursement purposes.

International Classification of Functioning, Disabilities, and Health (ICF): A framework for evaluating and classifying consequences of disease endorsed by the World Health Organization.

interrater reliability: The ability for multiple raters to obtain a consistent score on repeated attempts.

intervention: Care provided to a patient or client by a physical therapist or physical therapist assistant that includes coordination, communication, and documentation; patient/client-related instruction; and procedural interventions.

intraclass correlation coefficient (ICC): A reliability coefficient; a measurement of an instrument's reliability or repeatability.

intrarater reliability: The ability of one rater to obtain the same score on multiple attempts; also known as test-retest reliability.

The Joint Commission (TJC): An organization that accredits hospitals, ambulatory health care centers, home health agencies, and other health care organizations.

late entry: A chart entry written after original documentation and other health care providers have also documented; can also be written when enough time has elapsed so that the date you are writing the late entry is different from the original documentation; the entry should be identified as a "late entry."

long-term goal: *See* discharge goal.

maintenance: Services that can be provided by a nonlicensed individual, including the patient himself, a family member, or a caregiver who has had some training from a skilled professional. Maintenance services are not reimbursed by Medicare or many other third-party payers.

malpractice: A bad, or unskillful, act performed by a physician or other professional provider that injures or causes harm to a patient or client; includes the failure of an individual or group to follow the accepted standards that have been set forth by their respective profession(s). Includes willful, negligent, and ignorant malpractice.

managed care: A type of health care in which an insurance company (or third-party payer) maintains some control of costs and use of services and/or benefits.

medical diagnosis: The label assigned to the patient's injury, disease, condition, or illness.

medical necessity: As defined by CMS, medical necessity is a procedure and/or intervention that is appropriate and needed for the diagnosis or treatment of a medical condition; is provided for the diagnosis, direct care, and treatment of a medical condition; meets the standards of good medical practice in the local area; *and* is not mainly for the convenience of the patient or health care provider.

Medicare: The federal health insurance program for individuals (1) 65 years of age and older who are receiving or eligible for social security retirement benefits, (2) younger than 65 years with certain disabilities who meet the Social Security Act's disability requirements, and (3) with end-stage renal disease.

Medicaid: A joint federal and state program that helps with medical costs for individuals with low incomes and limited resources.

minimal clinical important difference (MCID): A value that represents an important, clinically significant change that the patient also perceives as beneficial.

Nagi framework: A conceptual framework written by Saad Nagi linking component of pathology, impairment, functional limitation, and disability.

narrative note: A documentation format in which pertinent information from the patient encounter is written in paragraph format.

National Center for Medical Rehabilitation Research (NCMRR) disability classification scheme: A conceptual framework for classifying pathophysiology, impairment, functional limitation, disability, and societal limitation set forth by the National Advisory Board on Medical Rehabilitation Research.

objective: The O: section of the SOAP note that includes measurable data or results of tests and measures, the patient's functional status, and interventions provided to a patient.

outcome: The end result of patient/client management; could also be the end result of an episode of care.

outcomes assessment: A patient (cohort) assessment designed to measure the end result of care provided; *see* functional assessment.

outcomes research: Research designed to scientifically measure the end result of patient/client management for a group of similar patients/clients; carried out in a clinical setting.

participation: The involvement in life situations, including performance of socially constructed activities such as work, school, or community involvement.

participation restrictions: Problems an individual faces while involved in life situations.

pathology: The interruption, or interference with the body's normal processes and simultaneous body efforts to heal itself or regain a normal state; often known as the actual disease or medical diagnosis.

patient/client management model: A model outlined and depicted in the *Guide to Physical Therapist Practice* describing physical therapist management of a patient or client; includes a description of examination, evaluation, diagnosis, prognosis, and interventions.

performance: Measured on the ICF evaluation scheme; includes the *extent* of the individual's participation restrictions or actual performance in his or her current environment. It is scored according to how much difficulty the individual experiences in life situations, such as performance of social skills (eg, work or community involvement), assuming the person wants to participate.

personal factors: Individual characteristics, such as age, race, gender, and comorbidities.

physical therapy diagnosis: A label assigned to describe the patient's movement disorders usually brought on as a result of the medical diagnosis; describes the relationship between impairment and function.

plan: The P: section of a SOAP note; indicates communication/collaboration, patient/client related education, and procedural interventions that are a part of the physical therapy plan of care.

plan of care: A plan describing what the interventions a patient will receive during the episode of care; includes the amount, frequency, and duration of services to be provided and may also include the expected final outcome(s).

practice act: A law, typically enacted by a state legislature, that governs the practice of a profession. All 50 states have practice acts that provide for licensure of physical therapists.

premium: A payment made to an insurance company to cover an individual under an insurance plan. Premiums are typically paid monthly. Many employers pay a portion of an employee's monthly premium as a benefit of employment. The insurance company pools the premiums received from a large group of individuals to pay the health care costs of those in the group.

primary care provider (PCP): A physician responsible for a patient's point-of-entry into the health care system. Some insurance companies require the PCP to be the patient's family physician. It can also be a general practitioner, internal medicine specialist, or in some cases an obstetrician/gynecologist.

problem list: A list of impairments, activity limitations, and/or participation restrictions that will be addressed with the physical therapy plan of care; found in the Assessment section of a SOAP note.

problem-oriented medical record (POMR): A documentation format organized according to the patient's problems; includes a patient-problem list that serves as a "table of contents" for the remainder of the medical record; subsequent entries include status and treatment for individual problems.

prognosis: Includes anticipated goals, the expected outcome(s), and may also include the ultimate plan for discharge; also includes the patient's potential for achieving his or her goals.

progress report/note: A special type of interim note that provides evidence for ongoing medical necessity of treatment; includes subjective and objective data and an assessment of patient progress including his or her status toward existing goals; also includes changes to the existing goals or plan of care, as well as justification for these changes.

prospective payment system (PPS): Medicare reimbursement provided to facilities (eg, hospitals and skilled nursing facilities) that is predetermined, or fixed, based on the patient's diagnosis and/or complexity.

protected health information (PHI): Individually identifiable information referring to an individual's medical history; previous, current, and future medical care; and billing and/or payment information, also known as individually identifiable health information. Also includes information that contains information that could potentially allow identification of the individual (eg, address, telephone and fax number, birth date, admission and discharge dates, voice recordings).

provider: An individual (eg, a physical therapist or physician) or an organization (eg, a hospital) that provides health care to patients.

reassessment: A regularly occurring part of the patient's episode of care during which the PT examines the patient's subjective and objective status to determine if further skilled care is medically necessary.

reevaluation: A separately payable services performed by a physical therapist when the assessment indicates a significant improvement, decline, or change in condition or functional status that was not anticipated. Formal, thorough, complete records of the patient's status, including tests and measures from the initial encounter, any additional tests and measures, record of new developments or problems the patient may be having. Includes specific progress (or lack thereof) toward goals stated on the plan of care. Can also occur within a required time frame dictated by law, a payer, or facility policy.

regulation: A rule established by a governmental agency that has been granted such authority by Congress or a state legislature.

reimbursement: Payment made to a health care provider from an insurance company, or other third-party payer, after being billed for a service provided to a patient.

reliability: The repeatability, or consistency, that an instrument or rater is able to measure a variable.

resource utilization group (RUG): The classification system used by Medicare to determine payment for care in skilled nursing facilities. Each patient in this setting is classified into 1 of 53 different RUG categories based on the types and intensity of services required to care for the patient. The skilled nursing facility is paid a daily rate to care for the patient; the daily rate is adjusted to account for the patient's RUG category.

responsiveness: The instrument's sensitivity to change.

review of systems: *See* systems review.

secondary insurance: Additional or supplemental insurance carried by a patient. The secondary will typically cover additional costs not covered by the individual's primary insurance.

short-term goal: An intermediate step to the patient's established discharge or outcome goals; a stepping stone to the discharge goals.

skilled care: A type of health care given when a patient needs management, observation, or evaluation by trained nurses or rehabilitation staff; also includes care that requires the unique judgment and/or skill of a trained individual for both safety and effectiveness.

skilled nursing facility (SNF): A freestanding facility or facility within a hospital, nursing home, or rehabilitation center that provides skilled medical, nursing, or rehabilitative services to patients. Examples of skilled services include intravenous injections, oxygen, feeding tubes, wound care, and rehabilitation (http://www.cms.hhs.gov/manuals/cmstoc.asp).

SOAP note: A documentation format that contains information arranged according to the headings S:, O:, A:, and P:, or subjective, objective, assessment, and plan, respectively.

standard error of the measurement (SEM): Quantification of the reliability, given in the same measurement units as the original measurement.

state practice act: A state's regulation of licensed professionals. Usually defines the educational requirements, licensure requirements, scope of practice, acceptable service delivery, and continuing education requirements.

subjective: The S: section of the SOAP note; information regarding the patient's status/condition provided by the patient, a family member, or a caregiver; includes the "history-taking" portion of the examination.

systems review (*or* review of systems *or* ROS): Part of the data collection procedures during a physical therapy examination; includes a gross review of body systems and measuring vital signs; used to guide decision making as to what tests and measures should be performed during the remainder of the examination.

test: A procedure or set of procedures that is used to obtain measurements (data); the procedures may require the use of instruments.

tests and measures: Specific standardized methods and techniques used to gather data about the patient/client after the history and systems review have been performed.

third-party payer: The insurance company or other health benefit plan sponsor that pays for medical services provided to a patient. The patient and the health care provider are considered the primary two parties.

treatment note: A type of interim note used to record interventions provided and serve as a record of what was billed; not intended to prove medical necessity.

validity: The degree that an instrument or rater measures the variable that it (or he or she) intends to measure.

World Health Organization (WHO): The directing and coordinating authority for health within the United Nations system. It is responsible for providing leadership on global health matters, shaping the health research agenda, setting norms and standards, articulating evidence-based policy options, providing technical support to countries and monitoring and assessing health trends (http://www.who.int/about/en/).

FINANCIAL DISCLOSURES

Dr. Mia L. Erickson has no financial or proprietary interest in the materials presented herein.

Dr. Ralph R. Utzman has no financial or proprietary interest in the materials presented herein.

Ms. Rebecca McKnight has has no financial or proprietary interest in the materials presented herein.

Index